T0229983

MEDICINE IN
METAMORPHOSIS

TAVISTOCK

MIND & MEDICINE
In 6 Volumes

MEDICINE IN METAMORPHOSIS

Speech, Presence and Integration

MARTTI SIIRALA

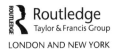
Routledge
Taylor & Francis Group

LONDON AND NEW YORK

First published in 1969 by
Tavistock Publications Limited

Published in 2001 by
Routledge
2 Park Square, Milton Park, Abingdon, Oxfordshire OX14 4RN
711 Third Avenue, New York, NY 10017

First issued in paperback 2014

Routledge is an imprint of the Taylor and Francis Group, an informa business

British Library Cataloguing in Publication Data
A CIP catalogue record for this book
is available from the British Library

Medicine in Metamorphosis
ISBN 0-415-26462-6
Mind & Medicine: 6 Volumes
ISBN 0-415-26512-6
The International Behavioural and Social Sciences Library
112 Volumes
ISBN 0-415-25670-4

ISBN 13: 978-1-138-86747-5 (pbk)
ISBN 13: 978-0-415-26462-4 (hbk)

Medicine in Metamorphosis

Speech, Presence, and Integration

Martti Siirala

TAVISTOCK PUBLICATIONS
London · New York · Sydney · Toronto · Wellington

This translation
first published in 1969
by Tavistock Publications Limited
2 Park Square, Milton Park,
Abingdon, Oxon, OX14 4RN
in 12 point Bembo

© copyright Martti Siirala 1969

SBN 422 73140 4

Originally published in Finnish under the title
'Peruskatsomustemme merkityksestä lääketieteessä: Konsultoivan psykiatrin havaintoja
puheenkehityksen häiriöistä' as a supplement to
the *Sosiaalilääketieteellinen Aikakauslehti* (Journal
of Social Medicine), October 1966, by the
Finnish Medical Association.

Translation by Jaakko S. Tola, M.D., and
Herbert Lomas, M.A.

Distributed in the United States of America by
Barnes & Noble. Inc.

Contents

Acknowledgements

I wish to thank most warmly all the permanent and temporary members of the phoniatric team – for their co-operation, for their encouragement, and for the abundant information they provided during our association. To Professor Urpo Siirala, M.D., who gave me the opportunity of working and carrying out research in the clinic of which he is head, I owe a special debt. I must also thank the Finnish Cultural Foundation and the Therapeia Foundation for the translation grants they provided.

I am extremely grateful to Dr Jaakko S. Tola, M.D., for executing the preliminary translation with such great devotion and skill. The final English version is the work of Mr Herbert Lomas, M.A., poet and formerly Senior Lecturer in English at the University of Helsinki. The process of articulating a 'new' approach is a painful one, and an essential share of this pain and difficulty has been suffered through by this friend of mine, and by the two of us together. He knows how grateful I am. Integration in speech presupposes enduring and persistent human presence.

Martti Siirala
Helsinki, September 1968

ERRATUM

Amendment to page 4, lines 5 to 13 inclusive:

... of speech. The human predicament at the base of any illness or deficiency cannot be really met through reduction and reification in isolation - cannot be meaningfully met. Encounter is required between man and his fellowmen. Reduction and reification – which are characteristic of what we customarily call 'natural science' – can never alone constitute a full encounter. They may prepare the ground, correct details and create certain necessary conditions for encounter. But the encounter must be allowed to take place, and have chances to become an unshortened, a human one and not become restricted to nothing but a number of measures based on medical objectivation – lest the response and the resulting encounter be real and not just seeming.

Preface

Dear Ronald Laing,

Judging from your books, you and I have encountered schizophrenia – in ourselves and others – in similar ways. I am taking it
for granted that schizophrenia is ubiquitous, or, in plain language,
that everyone is schizophrenic. Similarly, I am taking it for
granted that this is not, and cannot be, generally admitted: collective schizophrenia is not the subject of a bright collective
consciousness.

Interpersonal Perception – according to Marie Jahoda in her
introduction to your book of that title – 'approaches the full
complexity of human experience; it demonstrates that quantifica-
tion need not be limited to insignificant and artificially isolated
aspects of psychological phenomena . . .' These words touch a
sore point in the body of psychological science: a symptom, if
you like. You will understand what I mean because you are one
of the few who have undertaken to explore this symptom and
trace it to the *underlying disease process* in the *science* we profess. I
have used italics to indicate that the science does not merely treat
the disease: the science does not exist in some impossibly healthy
area outside the disease – in space, perhaps – but is immersed in
the human condition it is studying. The day has not only passed,
it has long since passed, when we could visualize a healthy
psychiatrist confronting a sick patient.

Nor is this diagnosis restricted to psychiatry. Psychiatry is part
of medicine, and medicine is sick because man is sick.

It is my belief that acknowledgement of this is a necessary
prelude to any realistic treatment of delusions. This belief is confirmed by the explorations you and your co-workers have been
undertaking; for you touch the sore point, the symptom of

disease in health, and in so doing open up new possibilities of therapy – new modes of experience, encounter, and thus of scientific research. Denial of a pathological condition, particularly if the condition happens to be in the doctor and controlling his concepts of health and disease, is not the best precondition for the emergence of new insights and knowledge. One of the consequences of such denial is in fact massive delusion; and one of the chief obstacles to therapy is the delusion that we have reduced diseases to mere object-things, entities that can be studied in isolation. I shall refer to this delusion as the delusion of reductive reification. As you will readily understand, I don't maintain that reification is in itself a delusion. It is reification as the pervasive approach, assumed as an autonomous position, in more or less complete unconsciousness that it is only one among many possible positions – it is this that constitutes a delusion.

Like you, I wrote my first book about schizophrenia: *Schizophrenia – des Einzelnen und der Allgemeinheit* (Schizophrenia in the Individual and the Community). This was published in German in 1961, and since my native language is Finnish I was immediately confronted by the problem, at all levels, of *communication*. Since this has some bearing on the present book, which is about speech dilemmas, perhaps I may explain a little about how the previous book came into being. It originated in two years of intense dialogue with one of the pioneers of the therapy of schizophrenia, Gaetano Benedetti. In that dialogue the language for articulating the experience itself, his and mine, was born. Between 1954 and 1957 I wrote the manuscript in German. The task was then taken over by a German poet, who struggled to make real German out of my home-made variety. In spite of all this labour, my book now seems more of a torso than a whole body. How shall I explain this partial failure? There seem to me to be two major reasons. First, the report was about a field of experience whose very existence as reality was, and still is, extensively doubted in 'scientific circles'. Second, to voice an experience of this sort the communicator needs to assume at least a minimum of readiness to listen and understand in his readers. Here was a basic existential difficulty aggravated by the distance of a foreign

2

language and situation. As a result, I tried to pour into this single vessel all my passionate experience of schizophrenia, disregarding the reader's legitimate demands for a restriction of the issues treated.

The basic dilemma of a child with speech disturbance is analagous to mine. Every child is a unique field of experience, an individual world. This world must reach out to other individual worlds in 'I–thou' relationships, and to the common worlds and world in 'I–we' relationships. In other words, a major dimension of individual human development consists of the possibilities of attaining reciprocal comprehensibility. How far can mutual verbal presence be reached between people? This depends on *fundamental non-verbal* conditions. Moreover, the 'common world', the world that receives each new individual into its midst, must fulfil certain minimum requirements. And the process of reception begins not with delivery, not even with conception. The reception has an immense historical dimension, which is, in principle, endless. The child is born into a family and a national and human network that extends across the generations. Only the most immediately recognizable meshes of this network are in the foreground. An example is the quality of parenthood that the father and mother have grown into – the couple that is creating, actualizing, the nest for the newborn. This nest must mediate at least a minimum of mutual human presence. It must provide some continuity of stimulus and response; it must make the child feel and think, and must recognize the child's feelings and thoughts; it must participate in the child's fundamental needs and provide the necessary exchange without which human development cannot take place. Otherwise no 'thou' can be formed, to be addressed in speech; and no 'I' can be formed to constitute a centre of speech.

This *minimum* requirement is equally demanded of the investigatory and therapeutic logopedophoniatric team. The team merely takes up the challenge, providing a 'second reception'. Society and the parents – or whoever *is* responsible for making the nest – delegate the task of assisting in the reception of the child with a speech disturbance. Whenever a child appears before such a team the first reception has been without exception a partial failure. The failure has manifested itself in non-integration: reciprocal verbal (or compensatory) comprehensibility has not been attained; nor has a reasonable degree of autonomy as a centre of speech. The human predicament at the base of any illness of deficiency cannot be met through reduction and reification – cannot be meaningfully met. *Encounter* is necessary – by man and his fellow-men. Reduction and reification – which are characteristic of what we customarily call 'natural science' – can never be a means of encounter. They many prepare the ground, correct details, create certain necessary conditions for encounter – sometimes absolutely necessary ones. But the encounter must be made, and it must be a human one, an integrative move, and not a medical objectification.

The kind of encounter meant here is most evident in the relation between a mother and her newborn child. Such concern and participation, mutual integration, is the only real way to fundamental redevelopment. And recovery, where defectiveness and illness are concerned, means fundamental redevelopment. Freud discovered this in the medical treatment of neurotics. Even more striking evidence has been provided wherever schizophrenia has been encountered without a primary reificatory position. Von Weizsäcker's 'anthropological medicine' – almost unknown in England, by the way – has demonstrated that these considerations apply to chronic bodily illness too. Von Weizsäcker's vast writings, and those of others inspired by him, particularly Kütemeyer, provide abundant insights into 'the full complexity of human experience' operative in bodily illness. A good deal of psychoanalytic interpretation, both of neurosis and bodily illness – the latter in terms of so-called 'psychosomatic' medicine – appears to be almost completely unaware of the problem of reification. Von Weizsäcker's work includes a profound analysis of the *delusion of an unlimited, primarily autonomous observer-position*, which is characteristic of our medical tradition. Another significant finding of anthropological medicine is the demonstration of the social pathology within individual bodily disease. The sick person is not an isolated phenomenon, and a truly therapeutic encounter reveals the shared common quality of the illness, not least in the therapist himself, who must acknowledge his share. The psychoanalytic term 'counter-transference' is a half-acknowledgement but does not sufficiently cover the experience.

Disturbances of speech development are a unique field for therapy in many ways: attention to the patient's needs, and to the needs of his immediate surroundings, demands the co-operation of vastly different professions. The membership of the International Association of Logopedics and Phoniatrics shows this. At its congresses – and this, I think, is quite unique – the medical profession is only one among many. Teams come from all over the world to these congresses, and, of course, the challenge of speech and voice disturbance is being met under the most varying conceptions of the nature of the task; yet the teams all have this variegated constitution. It is the existence of speech that accounts for this blessed multiformity. Speech is such that – in practice, at least – an attitude of neglect for the multidimensionality of the task could hardly be maintained. Insights into the nature and structure of human illness in general have almost forced themselves on these workers. And yet the insights have not penetrated into the general consciousness – least of all, perhaps, into the medical consciousness. One might have thought that the work of Kurt Goldstein alone – formulating universal anthropological insights from the specialized point of view of a neurologist involved with speech disturbance – would have been enough partly to remedy the situation.

In point of fact, then, my study is *an attempt to make a contribution to 'general pathology'*. To put it differently, I am trying to analyse some features of the basic structure of being ill or defective. My experience with a team encountering disturbances in the development of speech lent itself to this purpose 'quite naturally'. I have felt a sort of obligation to 'report' on the experience. In doing so I am aware of the vastness of the literature possibly relevant to the problematics here. This must be so in the very nature of the case. Equally clearly, a real immersion in this sea of literature would surpass the capacity of one man – and in any case drown the vital core of his thought. While many authors may justly feel that I am ignoring their contribution and neglecting the language of the dialogue, the ideas and approaches of certain others have become so integrated into my thinking that I find it difficult to quote them without doing so at impossible length. The latter include Luther, Kierkegaard, Freud, Heidegger, Binswanger, Bally, Benedetti, Boss, von Weizsäcker, Kütemeyer, Goldstein, and my brother Aarne Siirala, a theologian with whom I have continued a living dialogue over the last twenty years. It is significant that reciprocal comprehensibility between my brother and myself only began manifestly in adult life: this was after he had undergone a fruitful crisis through reading Luther's writings, and his insights made me receptive to the relevance of Freud.

I would, indeed, have good reason to quote extensively from my brother's writings. I shall content myself with a few ideas from his book *The Voice of Illness*. The immediate relevance to my own approach is easily seen. 'Man lives in continuous alteration between the symbolic word, creating oneness, and the diabolic, the splitting word.' 'The living word within a sick life situation has to be sought for under and through the distorted words.' The book develops the notion of illness as a message and a prophecy. He describes the resistances to the voice of illness, and the strategies for ignoring it, neglecting it, that are apparent in the histories of philosophy, theology, and medicine. He also examines the split between these dimensions of human experience in their encounters with illness and its message.

The pages that follow (mostly implicitly) concretely illustrate these notions. In particular, the split between theological, philosophical, and medical modes of encounter is, in my opinion, the chief reason for the preservation of the philosophically unsound delusion of an autonomous observer-position. Our whole view of illness has been fatally overshadowed by this. One manifestation of this delusion is that so little reporting of illness indicates our share in it. Yet the 'empirical material' of speech disturbances points in the opposite direction. The toughest resistances to exploration and therapeutic development are not in the isolated patient. They appear in manifold dimensions, both individual and collective. Sometimes, indeed, the most compact hindrance is found in a developmental deficiency in the child's speech. But the areas of hindrance may be altogether *other*. The chief obstacle may be the defective features of the nest. It may be the nest's insecure foundation in its society. It may be in certain attitudes of the parents. The greatest immediate obstacle may be in the family's social environment: in certain accepted and petrified attitudes towards speech and defectiveness. Again, certain traditional medical approaches may be the chief cause of stumbling and paralysis. Still more difficult obstacles may be legislative procedures that have little to do with medicine. Further, there is the team itself: transference is the essence of any profound therapeutic process; transference takes place on to the 'organism' formed by the team, producing tensions. In other words, the sick and healthy 'elements', the destructive and the constructive, *move through all possible dimensions of human existence and experience*. This idea is implicit in many authors' work, including yours, and it challenges quite radically the medical practice of 'locating' the illness or pathological process.

Since so much of this work is concerned with reassessing the impact of the subject–object relation on disease, I should perhaps emphasize my point of view. I am a consultant psychiatrist and chief of psychotherapeutic staff. I was working with a team in the phoniatric ward of the Department of Ear, Nose, and Throat Diseases of the University of Helsinki Central Hospital. At two-hour sessions, once a month, over three years, the entire ward and clinic personnel thrashed out in detail the cases that were most resistant both diagnostically and therapeutically. Several patients were being cared for month after month, one boy for a year. Some of the children were able to come several times for examination and treatment in the ward or out-patient clinic. I personally met only a few of the patients. Thus my picture of sixty cases is based on what came out of the team's meetings. I also studied the case histories of forty other patients. All these hundred cases are dealt with in a series of 150 patients studied by Aatto Sonninen (1964). The team included a phoniatrist, an audiologist-otologist, a psychologist with training in both psychometrics and psychotherapy, a speech therapist, a social worker with casework training, a kindergarten teacher, a nurse, a nursemaid, a hospital attendant, and a physical therapist. The purpose of the present book is not to consider all the case histories in detail. I am concerned with a shift in point of view and area of study. A case history is itself a reduction, a selection, an interpretation. It is a form of discourse, mainly narrative or descriptive, or a combination of the two. As such it is no less interpretative, no less pointed, than argumentation or exposition. There is a tone, an implication. These implications are significant for therapy, and in this book I shall examine them.

You will see that much of the book is concerned with the implications of 'reduction', 'mastery', 'control', and similar aspirations, and one may as well acknowledge here that the act of writing, the articulation of any communication, inevitably involves particular kinds of explicit and implicit reduction and aspiration towards control. Responsibility consists in acknowledging this with as much awareness as the particular researcher's development makes possible. Indeed, such awareness is a precondition for anything but the most mechanical kind of computatory labelling. A case history is the record of an encounter. It reveals as much about the doctor as the patient. Even an encounter with a plant will be very different for different individuals, depending on the range of interests, the philosophical standpoint, the particular concern, the capacity for awareness, and many other factors. A botanist, a forester, an artist, and a carpenter will not see the same tree.

The particular *gestalt* or configuration selected for recording in a case history is a simplification of a very complex phenomenon. We are not dealing with a tree but with a subjective being who is constantly totalizing the totalizer. The psychiatrist approaching a child patient is involved in a dialectic, a praxis. At the first impact the child sums up the psychiatrist (or the psychologist, the physician, or the nurse), and the child's behaviour depends on this totalization. The psychiatrist, in turn, is not dealing with a given object whose reified characteristics can be noted down botanically. He is also confronted by a totalization of himself, which is reflected in the child's eyes, symbolized by his gestures, implicit in every detail of his behaviour, from acute withdrawal, or 'autism', to the most active participation in joint play therapy or the dispensation of warm bodily affection.

Nor is the situation a static one. As the encounters proceed, the psychiatrist's fluctuating summings-up of the child, and the child's corresponding totalizations of the psychiatrist, are assimilated and modified. They are reflected on and find their place in the growing worlds of the two participants. Only drama could do justice to the fullness of living contact.

Nevertheless, the purpose of medical science is also to provide us with reductive controlling knowledge. It is to equip us with the power of more potent intervention in the situations of other people – our 'patients', who are not as passive as the word implies but are nevertheless judged, by themselves or others, to need such intervention.

The first step in the present study is therefore to present an appropriate reduction of the cases of five patients. These have themselves been selected from a much larger series of one hundred and thus initially constitute a reduction. I have not attempted to disguise the process of interpretation involved here. On the contrary, I have tried to make it explicit. In this way one may hope to avoid the presentation of implicit and largely unconscious assumptions and interpretations as if they were 'objective', or natural-scientific, facts.

These records of encounters, or 'case histories', thus constitute the initial interpretation of five significant human fates. The rest of the book consists of an exploration of the constellations involved and the requirements of adequate interpretation. Certain basic medical concepts are analysed: diagnosis, syndrome, aetiology, psyche, soma, etc., along with the preconceptions implicit in their usage. Certain new concepts are presented and applied. In sum, I have tried to uncover and analyse certain concepts of man and disease that are now being medically implemented. And I have tried to find new angles of vision, new areas of connection, to replace those that have proved fruitless. I have also tried to extend incomplete hypotheses.

Aware of the boldness of my task, I naturally look round for support. I would like to conclude this long letter by citing Kurt Goldstein, a significant figure in the development of research on neurological, psychopathological, and, in particular, speech development disturbances. The passage is from the preface to his book *Language and Language Disturbances* (1948), a fundamental work on the problem of aphasia.

Usually such an extensive study, demanding as it does so much knowledge and application of methods outside the usual medical field, is rejected as not medical, not physiologic, not empiric, and depreciated as philosophic. . . . In reply to such an objection I would like to refer to the general remarks made in my book *The Organism*, on this point. I came to the conclusion that the function of the organism could be understood only if we include that point of view usually called philosophic. When we approach the material with as unbiased an attitude as possible, and allow ourselves to be guided by the material itself and employ that method which the factual material dictates, the necessity of considerations customarily called philosophic may become apparent. The way in which these considerations have evolved from the material must show, indeed, that they actually belong to it. I should like to repeat the hope expressed in a previous volume: that it will be realized how irrelevant and little pertinent to reality are such lines of demarcation which are usually couched in the contradistinctive terms 'empiric research' and 'philosophic reasoning'.

On that note I should like to end,
Yours sincerely,
Martti Siirala

CHAPTER 1

Five Children with Disturbed Speech Development

I should like to begin by simply presenting a few concrete case histories.[1] They will, I hope, speak for themselves, as well as providing a concrete basis for the discussion that follows.

PENTTI

Pentti was nine. He spent altogether a whole year in the phoniatric ward. He came from a poor family in a remote country district, and he was hard of hearing. He and his younger sister, who also had defective hearing, had been more or less abandoned, left to their own devices. They had had few of the usual incitements to development and had remained enclosed, shut up, in their own worlds – Pentti more radically than his sister.[2] Clearly sheer continued poverty had helped to create the prevailing atmosphere of resignation. In such an atmosphere of despair the children's defective hearing was experienced as a hopeless wall, isolating the children from their parents. According to the father and mother, even the doctors had concurred in the despairing estimate of the situation. Pentti kept on running away from home, made no social progress, was troublesome in all sorts of ways at

[1] The text here closely follows the verbal and written reports of the team's psychologist, Pirkko Siltala.
[2] Pentti's eldest brother was the only one who developed without causing external intervention, but he was also an uncommunicative child. The next child in line died of pneumonia at the age of two months. Pentti too contracted pneumonia when he was three months old but just managed to survive. Pentti and his sister, aged six, did in fact appear to be very skilful in managing their bodies.

home, and became increasingly more difficult for his parents to bear. Thus there was a vicious circle: neglect and isolation led the boy to these reactions, but the reactions led to even greater rejection and isolation. As this went on the impenetrable circle increased round Pentti, for his behaviour gave the family a bad name in the village community. The parents then almost made him a prisoner in his own home, trying to prevent him from bringing shame to the family in the eyes of the village. This was a second imprisonment, for he was already a prisoner in his own being in the absence of speech communication.[1]

At the clinic Pentti appeared to be a veritable 'Kaspar'.[2] The strands that connected him to other human beings were of the slenderest. When he moved in a room, it was as if the people there did not exist for him – and he babbled oddly the whole time. However, the boy eagerly got his hands on anything mechanical. He would then quickly and skilfully pull it to pieces, and afterwards put it together again and make it work. What was the meaning of this? It was as if, deprived of human integration, he felt he had become a machine, in his dumb distress. Since the human organism had lost its humanity, and taken on its machine-aspect, humanity for him consisted in control of the mechanical.[3] Otherwise, his only way of being human, of visiting the human world, was destructive, bringing chaos, breaking objects and other children's toys, and striking other children.

Through play therapy, however, the world gradually began to open up other possibilities and dimensions for the boy besides

---

[1] When the members of Pentti's family were met in their home – after the present manuscript had been written – they appeared to be singularly impassive and slow to say anything. They gave an impression of helplessness, to an extent, but were not quite unready for combat where their two children were concerned.

[2] Kaspar Hauser (1812?–1833) was a German foundling raised in solitary confinement until picked up by police in 1828. 'Kaspar Hauser, whatever his prehistory may have been, is the prototype of the individual who has suffered from birth from impoverished relations with his cultural environment' (Alexander Mitscherlich, *Society without the Father*, 1969).

[3] Later Pentti returned for treatment with a phoniatric team in a new setting; this was also conducted by Dr Sonninen, however. In this phase of Pentti's therapy his machine-drawings gradually began to assume first animal and then human form – an interesting progression.

mechanical control. When Pentti was playing games with the play therapist, glimpses of an ability to share life appeared – if only for a fleeting moment. Sometimes the boy could even show an interest in this other person. For a long time in his games Pentti handled human figures as if they were merely things – simply objects among other objects. One day, however, man began to appear human in his games. Though hidden in a heap of wet sand, man began to emerge as man.

The child's most elementary forms of communication with his mother – and by implication with the world – were enacted in these games in many ways. His fuss about the hiding and giving of excrement came into this category. So did dramatic frameworks involving danger and destruction, of which there were many. Here in fact were dramatic presentations of the *destruction* actually experienced by the child. He was acting out the structure of his earliest relationships. In these dramas the child's responses to society were expressed: 'Look – my life has been destroyed, like this; and these things – all these things – these are what I need because I'm a human being.' Thus the child had an extremely differentiated intercourse with the play therapist: comprehension was possible, even though there was no vocal speech. Even the boy's utterances, mere noises though they were, gradually became increasingly complex and meaningful. Of course, no permanent social patterns of communication developed as yet.

As the communication with the play therapist very gradually opened out and grew in firmness, Pentti showed more solidarity in his behaviour towards others in the ward: there were signs of integrating tendencies. Along with this, the ward community began to experience him as increasingly more human. How was the boy experiencing his world at this time? His drawings began to show the possibility of the world's having friendly features, too: Pentti began to draw warm and cosy country homes in groups, with communicating footpaths and smoking chimneys. But – without exception – these miniature worlds were surrounded by water: they were on rafts!

As the world grew in intimacy and significance for Pentti, thunderous tensions were inevitable. Whenever situations reminded him of the rejection he had experienced, his reactions became violent. There were many occasions for this around Christmas time: the parents of all the other child patients in the ward came to fetch them home, but Pentti's did not. About the same time the boy's play therapist departed on maternity leave, and another person took her place. But the worst was yet to come. Isolated in his ward, because most of the other children were home for Christmas, Pentti lit a candle to celebrate his own Christmas and shut it in a cupboard. The message and the responsibility were complex and ambiguous, but some of the staff interpreted Pentti's message as 'bonfire' rather than 'celebration'. This danger, not legislated for in an ear clinic, his parents' distressed circumstances, and the lack of alternative forms of institution in Finland meant that Pentii had to be transferred to an institution for the mentally defective. The boy's hard luck, therefore, was to experience, as the phrases go, both 'early' and 'repeated' separation.

What about Pentti's case from the point of view of traditional diagnosis? One must recognize that both prolonged observation within the team framework and intensive and personal play therapy could only take such diagnosis some way. It was impossible to say, for instance, as yet, to what degree Pentti's hearing defect was central, perceptual, in character. In other words, one could not say to what extent his speech defect was aphasic. It was impossible to obtain adequately differentiated data concerning the boy's family, his mother's maternal condition during pregnancy, the delivery, his first year of life, or such matters as possible differences in the course of development between Pentti and his sister. Differentiated examination of his hearing was not possible as yet either. As to his general intelligence, the way he hustled around would suggest at least a good average level. Thus the total diagnostic picture remained at this level of incompleteness. But if diagnosis is considered as primarily a therapeutic signpost, the team did have adequate data for their purposes at the therapeutic stage then reached.

Pentti's Kaspar-situation became, through the communication achieved in play therapy, a therapeutic challenge to the entire team; even though the boy uttered no articulated speech, the *situation* was *eloquent* to the team. His play, his drawings, his elementary ways of seeking closeness, his vehement reactions when he remembered his fundamental frustration in some way – these were his pantomimic *language*; through this he *addressed* the team.[1] How far articulated vocal speech might have been able to develop as a manifestation and verification of his total *speech* (reciprocal comprehensibility between him and his world) if the therapeutic pattern of that time had continued without interruption, it is difficult to say. But clearly a decisively significant situation of reciprocal comprehensibility[2] was being set up and advancing: he was on the way to basic speech.

HEIKKI

When he arrived at the phoniatric ward Heikki was five years old. When less than one year old he had said 'Mother', 'Daddy' and 'give!'; but subsequently he started to use mere echo-speech, simply repeating phrases he had heard – sometimes recently but mostly long ago. As early as his second year the boy had started to batter his head against the side of his crib. He might bite himself.

[1] The team often discussed among themselves to what extent the boy might have an internal language, considering that even his expression through gesture was limited to the most elementary. His therapy then ran into a dramatic crisis, during which Pentti's play therapist became ill. The meetings were interrupted for five days. In the next play therapy session after this Pentti made a fish from plastic clay, gave it a baby rattle and – lulled it in his lap, crying the while.

[2] In Pentti's new therapeutic phase, consistently improving integration with the patient was achieved despite many obstacles. At the beginning of 1966, for the first time, the boy spontaneously used the sign language that had been taught him for communication. At about the same time Pentti showed signs of occasional tendencies towards taking another person's feelings into consideration. It was thus in the elements of mutual understanding that the therapeutic process still had to move. The way to recovery is certainly long, and it requires the continuing contribution of a large therapeutic team even after the most disturbed and trying stage of therapy has been worked through. Moreover, it is clear that the patient's future possibilities of development are decisively dependent on uninterrupted continuation of the therapy. This will decide to what extent the particular individual will ultimately be a productive member of his community, or alternatively a burden to it. (One might point out that in the therapy itself, too, the patient is already being a productive member of the community, if only for his productive effect on the team.)

Sometimes, too, but less frequently, his rage was directed against other people. For instance if chocolate were not popped into his mouth as soon as he woke up – this had to happen instantaneously, while he was still lying in his bed – his temper would be turned against others. This was a demand that had developed during his third year. It seemed to be implying: 'This, at least, you owe me!' Otherwise Heikki hardly asked for anything, to say nothing about *demanding*: he was content to remain in his own world. He never learned to be clean.

When the boy was one year old the family started building a house of their own, and this went on until the beginning of his third year. The building work completely consumed the attention of the father, and the mother tried to win the approval of her mother-in-law by earning money. She started to take work home and then devoted herself to it monomaniacally. When she brought her child for treatment, she asked: 'Could the disease have been caused by rejection of the child?' She said she had felt that all the time she devoted to the child, and not working for money, was 'wasted'. She had reached this degree of alienation from her womanhood and acceptance of her maternal rights.

From the first Heikki had been 'unwanted', and in some way the set-up implied that he was not approved of by his siblings, either. The father added: 'the child himself is not interested in others or things outside him'. He, the father, for his part 'had had no time . . . while the house was being built'. 'Life can't be lived on an emotional basis: one has to think of it in realistic down-to-earth economic and business terms. Security consists in having the economic conditions in order.' The father planned to emigrate, taking his family to some under-developed country, in order to find better facilities for economic advance. On the subject of his son's defects, the father also mentioned that Heikki was not able to look at television.

When he arrived at the ward the child was living entirely in his own worlds, and he was obviously having hallucinations at times. He had a way of repeating certain sentences he had heard long before. They seemed illustrative of the atmosphere in his family: 'Not in the train!' 'Don't bother me!' The boy could 'speak' all right, the 'mechanics' were there: but he was not addressing anybody. Actual echolalia (a sort of very elementary reciprocal comprehension and contact) could also be observed when Heikki was together with a three-and-a-half-year-old girl, whose dyslalia he imitated with virtuosity. Also, when Heikki put his hand into scalding hot running water, he could say 'Hot' – but he did not remove his hand from the water.

The boy did not respond when addressed. *Humming*, however, made him run to 'auntie's' lap immediately, even in the midst of a temper tantrum. Humming was evidently a signal of unhurried maternal presence for him: a symbol of union. Heikki became attached to 'auntie' fairly rapidly in the play therapy; he then attempted to defend his ownership of her quite heatedly in the ward. He *could* make demands, then, after all, although the ability was only articulable like this where the hope of experiencing permanent closeness had arisen.

At first Heikki became furiously angry, he bit and struck out, when the therapist repeated some of the boy's echo-speech. The therapist, it seemed, was trespassing upon Heikki's private world, where previously nobody had entered. Gradually, however, he began to repeat what 'auntie' had said; sometimes, even, he began to say things that had some actual content. Then this treatment was tragically interrupted. He had not yet reached the stage of *addressing* another person directly – but he was very close to it. He could, for instance, say (in the presence of the therapist, not his parents): 'I'm frightened', or 'Look, dad, look, mum!' His drawings became increasingly configurated, and once a truly startling move occurred: Heikki built a *house* (of building blocks) and offered it to his house-building father, who had come on a visit. The father said that it was 'the first sign the boy had shown of giving'.

As for Pentti, another Kaspar, the therapeutic games were quite primary: things were licked or brought to 'auntie's' lap; the boy put the therapist's finger into his ear; and so on.

Heikki could only be retained in the ward for two months. Then, due to the two-year waiting list, Heikki had to be moved elsewhere. He came from the other side of Finland, and it was impossible to arrange accommodation in Helsinki that would allow him to visit the hospital as an out-patient and also be reasonably satisfactory as a therapeutic milieu. Thus the treatment was unfortunately interrupted. The psychiatric hospital in Heikki's home district did not offer equivalent forms of therapy.

What does Heikki's case reveal about his speech development? Here was a boy whose early development was at first normal. It was in his second year, when he was left largely without the *attention* a child of that age would need, that serious trouble occurred: he became increasingly more autistic and, as regards speech, echolalic. This, as it were, involuntary rejection was part of his parents' autistic stance – the father's monomania about the purely economic 'standard of living', the mother's extreme uncertainty about her feminine role. These difficulties of the parents, disguised as economic concern, were at the root of the boy's speech difficulties. The boy's natural ability to make demands,[1] like his mother's, was readily paralysed by despair, and Heikki became separated and isolated from integration with other human beings: only very slender strands of connection and communication remained. The foundation of speech – the ability to make comprehensible exchanges concerning vital needs – was thus lost. His mother was unattainable – she could not be humanly reached: therefore nothing else could be reached. It was not worth while, not even possible, to say to his mother: 'Mother, I want something. Give it to me!' Naturally, then, there was no motivation for *further* speech either. He fell back on mechanical repetition, which expected no response. The boy's hearing and 'general sense' or intelligence were good; thus his echo-speech developed to a high level, but it remained a split-off phenomenon: it was *unconnected* with his personality centre, which, as a whole, had only meagrely formed. Readiness to return to differentiated

[1] The description does not attempt to provide an answer to the question of how decisive a role in this situation was played by, for instance, Heikki's eventually congenital or inherent, perhaps hereditary, impairment of the ability to make demands. The question, here, is of describing and analysing *the structure* of the illness-constellation of the patient. The important thing here is the form that questions regarding, for example, congenitality and heredity assume in the total explanation. There will be more on this later – pp. 34–42 and 66–75, for instance.

integration with others did, nevertheless, exist in the child, and it actually emerged, after initial resistance, in the play therapy. However, as with Pentti, we could not pursue this way through; or, rather, the door was closed for us.

EERO

Eero was six. He, too, like Pentti and Heikki, was a boy who had been separated early from his mother. And yet there are clear differences between the patterns of these three children. Pentti's human deprivation, his starvation of love and integration, was associated with his own hearing defect and his parents' economic distress, gloomy despair, and general hopelessness. Heikki's father, on the other hand, neglected his son in order to pursue a high standard of living; yet this was a manifestation of latent despair. And Heikki's mother neglected her son because her ability to defend her rights as a woman was easily paralysed. In the case of Eero his mother died when he was three years of age. Until then he had developed 'normally'. Even his speech had been 'normal, although somewhat delayed', according to the father. After the mother's death, Eero was cared for by his grandmother, in whose home the family had in any case been living.

As far as could be judged, however, this grandmother had very little maternal emotion to offer. Eero's father used a curious phrase in discussing her with the social worker: he referred to her as 'my grave'. It was clearly observable, too, that the father had remained suffocatingly dependent on the grandmother. After his mother died, Eero stopped speaking.

Interestingly enough, it was *not* for this absence of speech that Eero was brought for treatment. It was for chronic rhinitis. This was given thorough treatment at a ward of the Ear Clinic, and then one of the ward personnel began to consider Eero's failure to speak. The result was that Eero was transferred to the phoniatric ward, where he remained silent for the first week. During the transference procedures, however, Dr Sonninen did hear Eero speak. It was when the boy did not observe that the doctor was present, and what he was speaking to was the fish in the aquarium in the out-patient department. Eero spoke in a commanding, impatient tone: 'Go there – no: there!'

The ward impression of Eero was that his intelligence was normal, his hearing obviously close to the normal limits, and that he displayed no symptoms of cerebral injury. To begin with Eero was like a tiny, restless, peeping mouse. On the other hand, sadistic features soon became apparent in his relation to other children, and, simultaneously, he clearly invited punishment from adults.

During play therapy he gradually became more integrated with others, even in the ward, although there also occurred periods when he was locked up in himself and withdrew into solitude. With the female play therapist Eero went through elementary procedures, like Pentti and Heikki; but with Eero the transformation towards greater integration was more rapid. At first Eero tortured himself; then he tortured toy animals and puppets. Fairly soon, however, one of the animals became his special favourite, and it was not long before ordinary boys' games were accepted too. During treatment his querulous tone of voice disappeared almost completely. Next, explaining began to enter into Eero's speech, and he showed signs of understanding what had been said to him, although there was no clear response to being addressed. He himself could show the ability to address remarks towards other children, however, such as 'stop pushing!'

In the ward, Eero showed excellent skill in acquiring an 'auntie' for himself: he tamed a charwoman, who was considered irascible and treated him at first with cool indifference. Finally she became most warmly attached to Eero.

Eero's treatment was also threatened with interruption, but an opportunity was finally found for continuing the play therapy with Eero as an out-patient. Luckily the boy's home was not far away.

What was the nature of Eero's speech problem? Eero stopped speaking after the age of three, when he no longer had a mother, or a significant mother-equivalent. The world he had shared with his mother obviously had no continuity into the community beyond: it was cut off, a separate world, merely a sort of island in the itself sequestered, isolated, and constricting home of the grandmother. Eero's father had never been able to get beyond this isolated world. In a way, then, Eero's speech had remained something that only existed between his mother and himself. The father was remote on two scores: he was preoccupied with bread-winning and wrapped up in mother-dependence; so much so that he could not possibly respond to his son, be a pole of inter-communication. From his grandmother Eero could incite no response: since 'addressing' her was impossible, he did not even speak. Characteristically enough, the boy did discover a 'grand-ma' for himself in the ward; the armour of this lady he *could* penetrate – under the protection of the support he received in play therapy.

Thus the key to therapy in this case was an alternative mother. The problem was: where could a mother substitute be found for the boy – a permanent maternal supporter either in his normal environment or elsewhere?

ERIK

Erik was seven years old, a good-looking boy who spoke rapidly and indistinctly. He often left words unfinished, and his articula-tion was maladroit; at times, however, he articulated speech quite well. The boy gave an impression of intelligence. His behaviour in the ward was rather striking from the start; he was given to hard swearing, while excitedly trying to lift ladies' skirts.

Some degree of speech deficiency had occurred in the father's family. Prior to Erik's birth, his mother had had a miscarriage, and thereafter what was clearly a molar pregnancy. Erik was born somewhat later than term and was postnatally drowsy and cyanotic. The parents thought his early development normal, however, except for his vocabulary, which was slow to grow. The parents took Erik to the child welfare centre when he was two, because of his scant vocabulary, but they were reassured that he was normal. At the age of one and a half Erik suffered a so-called febrile convulsion, and he was otherwise frequently ill with infectious diseases during his second year. At the age of three to four years the boy manifested a kind of stammering, but it was not until he was five years of age that his parents noticed a general clumsiness.

Examination and observation in the ward revealed Erik to be intelligent. His motor function was maladroit, and he salivated. The EEG finding was 'Bradyrhythmia generalisata. Dysrhythmia epileptica subcorticalis centrencephalica'. Thus, from the traditional diagnostic point of view, the process here might seem to be a foetal or perinatal injury (or both), a cerebral injury acquired during the subsequent infectious diseases, or an inherited defect of the central nervous system. The case would seem to correspond to the symptoms of tachyphemia as listed by Arnold (1960), in which case the last-named alternative would be the relevant one.

Be this as it may, cerebral damage did not emerge as the main area of therapeutic conflict or offer the most solid resistance in his treatment. On the contrary, the defects in Erik's functional performance showed the greatest therapeutic plasticity. The most solid resistance and the most immediate front in the therapeutic conflict were elsewhere, in the parents' marriage situation. The key problem in the boy's disease pattern appeared to be here, in the tenuousness of the parents' relationship and in the immaturity that both partners displayed where decisions involving individual responsibility had to be made concerning their marriage. These points were also encountered in the boy's play therapy: they appeared as problems transferred on to him from his parents. During the half-year of his treatment in the clinic, Erik's parents were constantly teetering on the edge of separation or were actually separated. At one stage, while they again were living apart, the man was spying on his wife, ravingly jealous, threatening her with a knife. Thus the marriage situation, which should have been the basis of the boy's nest, his centre for growth, the nurture of his security, was a model of disintegration.

The boy's admission for treatment was clearly important for the parents' relationship: it gave them the permission and support they were apparently unconsciously seeking for pursuit of their *own* mutual clarification. This very necessary mutual explication and settlement they were unable to perform unsupported. Even with help the mutual explication remained indefinite, but at least something was set in motion and led the mother into continuous contact with the social worker. Erik's father, too, came – although irregularly – to talk with his son's therapist. It appeared that the man was immersed in Don Juanism of an almost psychopathic degree. Lying and boasting about a plurality of relationships with women, he was in despair, trying desperately to bolster up his male self-esteem. Disappointed in his experiences with women in general, he was paying it off upon his wife, on whom he was nevertheless extremely dependent. When he heard that his wife had a male acquaintance, he was driven to a psychotic reaction.

The wife's relations to men were unstable and stereotyped. She seemed to be married to her image of the male, rather than to the particular man who was her husband. Her image of man as mate was largely based on her mother's assessments, or on the assessments of others, anonymous mother-substitutes. Erik's mother displayed curious difficulties in grasping the total configuration, the unity of meaning, in a person's verbal communication. She found it difficult to get beyond the formal content of her fellow-human beings' words. Meanwhile, here too, the responsibility was shifted: without realizing it, she 'transferred the responsibility' for her personal reactions mainly on to certain imaginary rules. Such a woman is prone to be taken in by a man of deliberate charm and a boaster, and so it is not surprising she became the marriage partner of such a man. Meetings with the social worker, however, helped her to take a closer look at her situation, and gradually she began to be aware of the nature of her difficulties.

Arriving at the clinic, Erik was in a new kind of situation. Here the therapeutic team was prepared to take a therapeutic share in the responsibility for his whole nest constellation. People came from different directions to devote themselves to his personal treatment, intensive play therapy being the centre of activity. He responded by dedicating himself with the greatest intensity to the play therapy, thus 'treating himself'. This boy suffered from difficulties in concentration and difficulties with imagery and configuration; yet he was now able to dramatize his problems in the play therapy, and in doing so create dramatic imagery with the utmost concentration.

Of course, he had a lot to digest in the abrupt fluctuations in his parents' relations, and the marital comings and goings of his father. Erik was trying his best, struggling, to digest all this and preserve an acceptable picture of his father, an image that would be coherent to at least some extent. But all the time an agonized question was being revolved: 'What kind of a being is my father?'

During the play therapy Erik's clumsiness decreased. (Medical gymnastics clearly contributed to this too.) His visual perceptions improved as his image-making assumed firmer configuration, and the boy ceased to salivate. His speech became more intelligible, and cluttering and dyslalia at times disappeared almost entirely. Also, the erotization of his contact-making declined, and his association with the others in the ward became altogether more adequate.

The admission of the child's nest situation into the therapeutic process and Erik's integration with his fellow-beings in his immediate distress were taking effect: they were creating a situation of relevant reciprocal comprehensibility. Mutual understanding and integration were occurring between Erik and his fellow-beings. As a result, his speech defect, his general motor disability, and his difficulties in image-making pronouncedly lost their power to interfere with his communication and movement, although clearly the process was not complete.

Fortunately the shortage of beds did not terminate the treatment. The process was able to go forward ambulatorily, with Erik as an out-patient, for the mother continued to participate in the treatment, and the home was not far from the clinic.

LAURI

Lauri was three when his mother heatedly clamoured over the telephone that the boy must be taken into the hospital straight away, jumping the waiting-list. The reason? 'Lauri's making my husband nervous, and he's got an official party to celebrate his promotion in a few days!' With this kind of high-pitched peremptoriness she was trying to cover her insecurity as both woman and mother.

A paternal cousin of Lauri's father had a cleft palate. In addition, it appeared, the boy's mother had used a thalidomide product against insomnia during her pregnancy. Lauri was born with a cleft palate; later on, he was also found to have nasal septal deviation, inguinal hernia, and flat feet. No fault was observed in his sensory organs nor in his 'general sense', or intelligence. There were three previous children in the family. The father was a professional technologist, twelve years older than his wife, who was a university-trained business woman. Together they had created a high standard of living for their family. When the busy father, who was rushed off his feet, was, for once, seen in the ward, his hand was in a plaster cast: he had slipped on the parquet floor of his house. At the few and hurried meetings with the mother in the ward, she appeared to be very ambivalent about her own femininity. She said: 'I should have given Lauri away immediately. He's a total stranger to me. I only like girls. My husband and I, we don't like small children.' The questionnaire sent to the parents was completed by the mother in a rebuffing tone. There was no single mention that Lauri had spent the first thirteen months of his life in an orphanage. Asked about this, the mother replied that he had been apathetic in the orphanage, but well-behaved and cheerful. Taken back home from the orphanage, he certainly continued to be apathetic, but if he was left alone he shouted and threw things. In the mother's eyes Lauri was 'a strong, terribly self-willed character'. She said they were planning to send Lauri to a boarding school abroad as soon as he was seven.

Lauri's parents could not be brought into any kind of continuing co-operation in his treatment. The outlines of this tragedy of early separation thus remained merely sketchy.

Lauri was found to be an exceptionally charming child, who soon became the pet of the ward and the out-patient department.

A great advantage from the point of view of his speech development was his fine sense of rhythm. (All the children in his family were known to be musically talented.) The first contact with the boy proved easy, though superficial, Lauri making no distinctions between degrees of acquaintance and familiarity. He was observant and active, though apathetic and unresponsive at times. Following adenoidectomy, he stopped speaking entirely for some time and started babbling. When his sister, who had nursed him, departed from the ward, Lauri cried bitterly; when his mother arrived he reacted with regression of speech.

The overwhelmingly central question for therapy was: where can we find a nest for Lauri in which he can develop? True, his thirteen-year-old sister had taken care of him, and Lauri was very attached to her – but permanent fulfilment of his need for parents still remained an unsettled problem.

The deficiencies in Lauri's speech ability were clearly associated with his cleft palate, but only in a limited way. A *fundamental* prerequisite for speech development, on the other hand, is a home that will accept the child to at least some extent: and this was lacking. The boy's visible and audible defectiveness was the final and insurmountable barrier for the parents: they could not step beyond this threshold, for even without this they were ambivalent about parenthood and were trying to escape from the whole problem, and from their despair, through a desperate preoccupation with a high standard of living. In Lauri's case, too, then, the most solid resistance to solution and treatment was not encountered in the 'objectively' observable mechanical defectiveness of the patient, but elsewhere.

CHAPTER 2

Constellations

Speech, in its various forms, manifests, realizes, and develops a central feature of man's being: his capability of reflection. Man's reflectibility, his self-mirroring in consciousness, constitutes human intelligibility: man's intelligibility for himself and for his fellow-men. Speech is thus crucial for man's understanding of himself, but it is also self-expression and a way man has of inhabiting his world. According to Heidegger, language and speech are the 'dwelling' of being: the 'home' in which man lives. ('Die Sprache ist das Haus des Seins. In ihrer Behausung wohnt der Mensch.' Heidegger, 1947, p. 5.) The meaning is twofold: language is built as a dimension of man's being; and language itself builds the being of man. Through speech – vocal speech, writing, gestures, hearing, lip-reading, meaning, understanding – mutual integration occurs: through speech man integrates himself with himself and others, with the continuity of his own history and the history of his family, his country and mankind, with culture and the world, and with being in general.

This process of integration is prolonged – long-range in nature. The basis of integration – and therefore the basis of mutual intelligibility and of intelligibility to oneself – is presence: the presence of man to man, of man's being to man's being: the presence of the human mode of being in general, and the presence of individuals who are each unique manifestations of man's being. The presence of a baby to its mother – where a mother is aware of her baby, aware that her baby's being and expressions

27

are addressed to her and touch her inner being – is perhaps the most immediately obvious manifestation of the presence of one human being for another. Yet even this is by no means a straight-forward situation without preconditions. The growth and maturing of a woman for motherhood demand at least certain minimums of human time, space, and nurture. Pregnancy, delivery, and the framework of receiving and caring for the new-born (a framework here called 'the nest') must fulfil certain basic prerequisites concerning human security, if the presence of the child to its mother is to have an opportunity of manifesting itself. The mother is thus made possible by a community, is an embodi-ment of the values and gifts of the community. And in herself the mother – together with her spouse, provided there is one – is receiving the child on behalf of the community. It might be said that the community, first in the shape of the mother and subsequently in the form of both parents, is thus encountering the presence of the child, identifying him and taking him into account in various ways and degrees. In such ways and in varying degrees the community thus acknowledges – or fails to acknow-ledge – the presence of the child (and later, the adult) as building material, as a human component for the creation of its own human reality, the human community.

Presence is the foundation of speech. In order to speak to you I must be present to and for you: I must in some way touch something in you – at least, if there is to be a permanent basis for speaking communication. For a child, the foundation of learning speech is his presence to his mother, to his parents, or their substi-tutes, and, through them, to the community of men in general. The later and larger presences, the presence of *other* men experi-enced as the presence of 'fellow-men', the presence of the world to him, the presence of being – even the presence of his *own* being – are built on the initial experiences of presence: they grow out of the way the child experiences his own presence to his parents, his community, and the world. The specific ground for an individual's speech and speaking is the history of the nest and the subsequent phases of his own presence.

If these considerations are applied to the childhoods described earlier, 'constellations' of different structure can be observed. The full meaning of the word 'constellation' will gradually emerge from the discussions that follow.

For Pentti, the innate (hearing) defect signified a particular impediment in learning to express his presence as a vocally articulate person, to be present as human speech. In the economic distress, apparent isolation, and resigned existence of the parents, the deafness was enough to create a block between the child's presence and a living response from the parents.

As for Erik, the partly congenital and partly acquired defect in some dimensions of the control of the general sensory and motor performance (associated with the cerebral function) did not in itself lead to complete discouragement or a rejection in the parents' attitude. The nest as a whole was threatened by disintegration. The parents had married partly in an attempt to repair the helplessness they both evinced; in consequence their relationship was very flimsy, insecure, unintegrated, and quarrelsome. The presence of the child was in fact identified, but only amidst continuous controversy, insecurity, and instability. This instability extended into the general sensory and motor performance of the boy.

Lauri, on the other hand, had no congenital sensory defects; nor had he any weakness of control in the general sensory and motor performance. Instead he had a defect that disfigured both his appearance and his voice: a cleft palate. In the parents' distorted life – for it *was* distorted, however inconspicuously by conventional standards – *this* blemish motivated a disregard, even a rejection, of the child's presence. Evidently, the most significant factor in the disease constellation was this distortion in the parents' existence, and the accompanying 'deafness' to Lauri's presence. At all events, cleft palate does not in itself lead to elective mutism.

Heikki, for his part, had insufficient time to stabilize his speech-ability before a phase of the nest began in which his presence was submerged beneath his family's monomania about house-building. His ability to demand what he needed – which was already rather weak – thus lost an important mode of expression, the vocal one: vocal speech did not assume its natural function and most elementary task. On the contrary, his speech lapsed into the position of an echo, containing the mere attenuated reminiscences of an address and answer situation.

In the case of Eero, the only response to his presence was in his mother. When she died, the motherless boy was abandoned to the situation in which (perhaps 'because of' which?) she had died: he was left in the house of the father's mother, where the family lived. The father called his own mother his 'grave': he could not get away from her, out of her, into life, and become sufficiently independent of her to form a nest of his own. Thus, until his mother died, Eero had a nest that was an isolated island disconnected from the father and from the rest of the community. When his mother's death disintegrated this nest, there was no other there or available: the boy's presence was deprived of reception; there was no continuity between him and the community, and Eero became dumb.

II DIAGNOSIS AND ITS DIFFERENTIATION

At least in the cases briefly analysed above, a diagnosis based on symptoms and syndromes would help us very little, for it would not reveal the facts of the broader disease constellation. In psychiatry an attempt to overcome this type of deficiency has been made by differentiating the diagnosis and dividing it into different groups. Such groups might be: (1) descriptive, symptomatic diagnosis; (2) dynamic diagnosis, relating to personality dynamics; and (3) genetic diagnosis, or the history of the origin of the disease. In child psychiatry, in particular, the problematic nature of symptomatic diagnosis has long been noted. Anna Freud's team attempted to improve the situation by developing a new diagnostic scale based on the degree to which the child's development had been affected.

How a diagnosis is formed and the nature of the diagnosis are, of course, largely determined by the goal of the diagnosis. Yet another factor in the situation is incomplete awareness of this. Traditional diagnosis is often performed with only partial consciousness that, in short, the nature of the diagnosis is fundamentally dependent on the mode of medical thinking, on the type of basic attitude in the diagnostician, on the concept of both disease and man, and on the purpose and application of the diagnosis. Where there is disturbance of speech development, the first orientating diagnosis is made *unprofessionally* – by the child and its parents. Again, at the preliminary medical levels, thorough investigation and therapy do not take place: the main aim of diagnosis is to determine the proper place for specialist treatment. If the place selected is, for example, the Clinic for Ear, Nose, and Throat diseases, there too the early diagnostic measures will have a similar function of determining where to delegate the problem. As the patient approaches the centre with final responsibility for examination and treatment, the diagnosis becomes increasingly part of the treatment: that is, the particular orientations of the various clinics have therapeutic consequences.

Often, too, diagnosis signifies an ultimate total conception of the medical case. If, however, the total conception (implying a total attitude) is simply that of the traditional symptomatic or syndromatic diagnosis, limitations are apparent: such diagnoses do not have the power to provide a general orientation regarding the disease constellation, which encounters one as a multiplicity of facts. This limited significance and value is, of course, sometimes decidedly useful: it may help us to know, for instance, whether an organ, or an entire organism, is in immediate danger; and if so, how; and whether particular strategic measures are needed to combat the danger. The case is different, however, if we are seeking to form a total conception of a medical case and ask what the functions and requirements of diagnosis are from this point of view. In that case the psychiatric diagnostics referred to above (and not confined to children) make an essential supplement and improvement, particularly where disturbed speech is concerned. Let us now examine a diagnosis composed of such elements, taking the case of Lauri as an example.

1. *Symptomatic diagnosis:* There is occasional mutism, nasal speech, and a tendency towards regression to infantile behaviour.

2. *Genetic diagnosis:* There is a possibly hereditary disposition to

cleft palate. The mother had had thalidomide medication, which possibly produced a traumatic effect on the development of the foetus. The child has a cleft palate, flat feet, and inguinal hernia. His parents have almost rejected him. The parents are very inadequate for parenthood, particularly where there is a need to accept a deformed child; they even have a conscious unwillingness for the task.

3. *Dynamic diagnosis:* The child can only speak and behave in accord with his age level and other presuppositions in conditions where he experiences himself as directly and continuously present to his fellow-men.

4. *Developmental diagnosis:* There is a severe degree of developmental disturbance, which is demonstrably reversible. The development of the situation (the prognosis is here organically connected with the diagnostics) will depend decisively on whether the elementary prerequisites for the child's development can be guaranteed – on whether a family substitute can be found, or at least progress made in this direction.

Clearly, such a group of diagnoses already reflects Lauri's true state to a considerable extent, since it clarifies at three levels: the total conception, the possibilities of orientation, and therapy. Naturally, this is not an automatic merit of a diagnostic scale, but if a multidimensional diagnosis is required, the diagnostic and therapeutic practitioners are apt to be more conscious of the nature of their task. The scale, with its classifications, is certainly too narrow to predict all the categories of man's being in which the diagnostics have to move. No scale should be regarded as sufficient: the diagnostics must, in fact, be flexible enough to develop into ever new dimensions, which means a perpetual rectification of prevailing diagnostic attitudes.

In the case of Pentti, for instance, the diagnosis should clearly include an explication of the social structures and pressures that encouraged the parents to become 'deaf' to their half-deaf son. His diagnosis should also elucidate why the team that accepted him for examination and treatment was unable to pursue its task beyond a certain limit. Part of Pentti's diagnosis is why the team could not cross a certain threshold.

It might well be asked, however, whether considerations such as these truly belong to the diagnosis and systematics of diseases in general. Are they merely casual factors having nothing to do with the 'disease process as such'? This question will therefore be discussed in the following section.

III BASIC STRUCTURAL
COMPONENTS OF DISEASE CONSTELLATIONS

I shall first attempt an answer to the question posed at the end of the preceding section and then seek an orientation for the associated problems. First, as already pointed out, man's speech is an eminently supra-individual occurrence. While he is speaking, man is never a mere individual: he is always being a fellow-man as well – even when he is speaking to himself. Speech is among the most obvious dimensions of mutual integration between human beings. Only for quite limited purposes is it reasonable to consider speech as merely an individual matter; otherwise the procedure is arbitrary. Pages 106-7 of the present text, in analysing the concept of existing, indicate how man's whole being is always, from a certain point of view, joint existence: man is a fellow-man. (Man's being is always relationship to himself, as well; and it is also presence in the world and the universe.) A physiology and pathology which try to confine their study to *individual* behaviour – to a behaving individual in man – and to the structures and functions that can only be isolated in thought are proving inadequate as an exclusive research attitude. Among other evidence, the children's lives in the first chapter of this book show the need for more multidimensional study.

A survey follows of a few basic structural elements of disease constellations, facts encountered in conditions of disturbed speech development. These will include the following: our latent concepts of the community and of the body, and the attitudes that result from these; the distortion of oligophrenia through discrimination, and its congealment through latent despair; haste –

the feeling that there is not enough time for existence – transferred from the community to the individual and thence to an organ; exaggerated demands for obedience. A person's potentialities and presence can be expressed in all these modes of being and concern. A dominant point will be the following: the part that the struggle between hope and despair plays in forming disease constellations and, one must emphasize, medical doctrines and other communal hypotheses concerning disease.

(a) As modern communities have evolved, there has been an increasing recognition of the equality of men in extending dimensions. A man's most manifold needs for development, treatment, and care have been acknowledged. And yet, at the same time, ever new forms of discrimination have developed from century to century. Rejection, contempt, depreciation, and implicit, or indirect, denial of another's elementary rights now occur less and less openly; for discrimination has, in principle, begun to be much more generally disapproved of and put aside.

Yet the *conception* underlying the separation from ourselves of those we condemn remains. This conception is our conception of the human community: what it is like, and what its structure and nature are. The conception is mainly latent: it is neither expressed nor recognized, yet it prevails. If this conception is operative in us, latently or otherwise, we start from the following assumption: any defectiveness or anomaly – even any difference – does not belong to the 'community proper': it is, as it were, primarily 'outside'. Faults, defects, and diseases do not belong to the community 'proper'. The community, our life in common, with its institutions, is imagined as healthy in itself, and at most impeded by various circumstances and disadvantages.

Apparently, too, our implicit premise is the assumption that every human individual should normally possess abilities that are, at least broadly speaking, adequate for independent existence; or rather, that he should have the making of such abilities. Such a reduction of man and his basic needs is only possible through primary objectification of him, confining the scrutiny within a short-term perspective. Only in this way can we fail to observe the actual multidimensional network of preconditions for being a man and growing into a man.

Man also seems to have a special interest in dispelling from his mind certain of his fundamental dependences. He wants to forget about his dependence on the creation, on other men, on the jointly created total mental atmosphere, and on organic integration as a community, having both contemporary and historical dimensions. And yet the most commonplace everday experience reveals our dependence on one another: the realization of individual projects essentially occurs through the process of mutual integration. Individuals certainly do differ fundamentally in their talents; yet the individual's talents do not exist in isolation: they depend on those of other people. These two facts – individual differences and interindividual dependence – belong structurally together. The individual's talents and the community's talents and potentialities depend essentially on recognition of integration: what happens to the talents depends on how far man's fundamental general dependence and men's interdependence are given recognition.

In spite of this, it is customary for an individual labelled with some deficiency, defect, or disease to be experienced as *exceptional* in his fundamental dependence on others and on life in general, though this works crucially against the person in question and against his development, in particular, which is associated with the defect. It thus finally works against the community as well, which is ignoring a dimension of integration that is organic to its own reality.[1]

[1] The problem of potentiality and talent may be illustrated through the following picture: if mankind possessed, for instance, 10^{20} different potential talents, the Finns would probably have 10^7 and Finnish individuals would each possess 10^2 to 10^4. Studies do not appear to exist where the talents of various social units (beginning with the family) would be investigated as to how the talents develop, are selected or discouraged in different communities. It seems to be the case that genetic studies have so far taken the individual as the sole type of unit. Is there, however, no motivation for studying the frequencies of the various talents and defects in a whole context? Or how the talent and defect profiles of individuals are composed? Or how these profiles appear when viewed against the background of different social units and mankind's total resources of talent? (Of the latter, of coures, merely the principal outlines could be established.) Would it not seem

Defects and disabilities are one thing and variation is another, although it is not easy to draw a definite line of demarcation. After all, the variation over the whole range of the human community implies that each individual will have at least some disabilities and defects. In addition, everybody dies: every individual eventually encounters death, travelling along a specific path of his own to the general fate; and the circumstances of his death always bear some relationship to his potentialities, that is also to his genotype. In some sense, then, it is absolutely universal to be defective, normal to become ill and die. And yet, even in medicine, there is a tendency to maintain a dominant image of the intactness, the freedom from defect, the health, of the normal individual, who is thus absurdly endowed with immortality. In this way the ubiquity of debilities, disabilities, defectiveness, illness, and gradual and total bodily death are effectively denied. Society is, in fact, dominated by the latent delusion of an ideal community. One result of this is the pattern of problem-setting in medical research.

For one who works within the framework of this delusion of an ideal community, the dominant question that is likely to emerge is: how does the defect of this individual, or that individual, constitute a deviation from the norm? But if the 'normal' individual is imagined as largely undefective, 'healthy', and in principle independent of his fellow-men, and if the life in common, with its institutions, is assumed to be neutral, then a crucially distorted background has been created for encountering a defec-

called for, too, to investigate the polarity of different talents and aggregates of talents, not only in individuals, but between individuals and between different types of social unit?

Concerning the cases of retarded speech development he studied, Sonninen remarks: 'All groups contain a comparatively large number of features suggestive of brain damage, lack of linguistic talent, "genic anomalies" and psychic disturbances. In patients with defective hearing such traits are less common to a statistically significant degree, but even among these patients the number is remarkable. Despite the most careful investigation, the results are relatively meagre. One reason for this is that data about the occurrence of corresponding symptoms in people in general are lacking.' Sonninen also cites Gesell and Amatruda, who consider that 'every child born alive has been subject to the risk of general brain damage'.

tive individual. If, in fact, imperfections and defects do characterize the whole community, if they are part of the community's
problems of existence, then we inevitably distort an individual's
defect by regarding it as confined solely to the one person. Yet
this, it seems, is what occurs when a patient is examined in isolation, or if his environment is arbitrarily circumscribed, or if it is
supposed that certain 'evidence provided by the senses' gives direct
information concerning the nature and true configuration of the
defect. Is this not an implicit denial that the total configuration
of the defect might extend to the community? And must not the
'community' be understood as including those habitual attitudes
and ideas within whose limits we tend to act – and act, too, upon
the very defects in question?

Later in this study I shall try to demonstrate that close scrutiny
of the investigational and therapeutic team's reactions to a certain
patient is an essential component of the diagnostic work. Such
scrutiny can, in fact, be seen as an opportunity to explicate the
very communal factors that are structural elements of the patient's
defect constellation. But, in point of fact, the community will not
readily acknowledge these factors as its own; it will be disposed
to encounter them only as located elsewhere – in the individuals
that the community has identified as defective. Perpetuation of
this attitude, however, is something that the therapeutic and
investigational team cannot afford.

As already mentioned, a thoroughgoing attempt is constantly
being made to reject the ubiquity of death from the communal
consciousness (and from the responsible formation of attitudes in
general). This involves efforts to reify, objectify, and 'place' death:
death is, among other things, the immutable, the irreversible, the
immovable; we wish to manœuvre it into a position where we
can 'have' it as nothing but defects, disease, and destructive influences. The 'death-content' of our own mode of being – and the
particular behaviour this involves – remains hidden from us.
When 'death' manifests itself in terms of sheer hopelessness, our
own despair, we dare not experience it at all. We must locate
it anywhere we can. This locating and avoidance form one
dimension of the prevalent communal depression, from which the

clinical depression of individuals derives.[1] Through communal depression various kinds of defectiveness set up associations with death and are experienced as 'death': this is one aspect of the community's unacknowledged death-worship. I would use the term 'death-worship' for the prevalent institutionalized hopelessness, which is also rejected from consciousness and denied.

The simultaneous abjectness before and rejection of death make it difficult to include relevant questions in the problem-setting. Is a certain defect possibly, for instance, the reverse aspect of some potential talent? Despair almost disables us from asking this kind of question. Hope is necessary for certain types of thinking to be conceivable: we cannot see any good in pointing out that a defect's total configuration extends into the community, unless we can conceive that *new life* might possibly emerge out of bringing this latent 'death-content' into communal consciousness. Or if some new and challenging integration between the individual and the community is called for, it is hard to accept that some long-prevalent communal structure has to *'die'* away, in order that something new and more viable may replace it. We find it impossible to believe that death might contain new possibilities of life; thus any suggestion of death is more than we can bear. In fact, this attitude is, I find, one of the 'doctrines of despair' that are prevalent in the community and manifest themselves in the clinical depression of individuals.

The 'placing', the locating of 'death', performed from a standpoint of desperate but disavowed fear, amounts, however, to carrying death into effect. True, the act of fixing the location of 'death' does afford some relief: we can escape from encountering *some* distress. But what did Lauri's parents, for instance, achieve by this? From what could their attitude possibly extricate them? They lived as if the ultimate disaster (the threat and realization of death) existed *in the boy's defects*. Their fanatical struggle for a 'higher standard of living' seemed to be an attempt to persuade themselves that some aspect of their life might hold richness and

[1] This is explicated in my articles 'Schizophrenia: a Human Situation' and 'Self-creating in Therapy'.

wholeness; they were disguising their actual 'poverty' and disintegration; these were facts they had difficulty in facing with any degree of hope. But now, by locating 'death' in the defectiveness of the boy, they only aggravated the defectiveness, for he was thus left without many of the preconditions and incentives for development that a nest should contain.

Despair, reverence for the power of death, is highly contagious; it also has the property of becoming, gradually and inconspicuously, 'self-evident', unchallengeable, thus losing its painfulness. Resignation sets in. The resignation resulting from repressed fear of death becomes institutionalized *medically*: it takes the form of erroneous hypotheses and structural features of the medical institutions and the health service as a whole. Nor were we, the team of the phoniatric ward, exempt. We sometimes got an insight that the latent resignation prevalent in the patient's disease constellation was affecting ourselves and about to lead us into quite inapplicable assessments of the situation and the possible solutions.

An example of the inadequacy induced by despair would be the following. A girl aged three and a half had both her external ears deformed. She was somewhat hard-of-hearing and shy. Her parents considered her to be mentally retarded. For them this implied a hopelessly global defect in their child. In the ward, however, the girl proved most intelligent. True, she did not speak much, and then only to a few persons whom she had selected, but on the other hand she proved quite capable of development, even in speech.

The cases of several other patients revealed that a defective child's shyness reflected the family's tolerance or intolerance of defects, which in turn reflected the attitudes of the wider community. The shyness was not primarily a characteristic reaction pattern of the child (although a child's shyness *can* be that). Even in the worst case, the implication is that the burden of suffering for a defect that is actually communal has become the sole responsibility of the individual who is experiencing the agonizing shyness.

Discrimination may thus throw the burden on to the deficient child, but the discrimination is not always experienced directly in the family. Such discrimination may only appear indirectly.

How discrimination is indirectly acknowledged and influential is shown by the family of a girl aged five and a half with sub-mucosal cleft palate and nasal speech. She was a very intelligent child, capable of good contacts, and her family constellation was in many aspects solid. Nevertheless, the girl's speech was less developed than would be expected. There was a clue in the parents' constellation. Apparently, the father of the family also had a cleft palate, and he had opted out of many responsibilities for speech: he had learned to avoid the risk of discrimination by leaving matters requiring speech to the mother. Thus the parents had provided a model of resignation for the child – speechlessness in the presence of discrimination. This created the atmosphere surrounding speech, even though the child escaped *direct* experience of discrimination within her own family circle.

Incidentally, the acoustic configuration created by *nasal* speech is clearly a particular aversion of the community, for some reason. The extent varies with different communities, of course, as nasal speech enters into the ordinary speaking practices of certain peoples. With nasal speech the main factor is certainly not defectiveness of the function: the trouble here is the 'aesthetic' overtone, the solecism in plasticity; we are bothered by the deficient integration of the total configuration. Fortunately, the discrimination surrounding the child does not always prove intractable or lead to rejection. It may fade away – when, for example, the child's parents become aware of the potentialities their child does have, and the potentialities of the whole situation. Such developments reveal the importance of hope. It shows that despair is at the basis of discrimination. With the emergence of hope discrimination loses some of its force.

For instance, a feeble-minded girl aged eight and a half, had a cleft palate and nasal speech. The parents had experiences of contact with the phoniatric ward, in which they were aroused from their resignation. When the girl was re-examined at the age of eleven, her condition had substantially improved.

If defects have *accumulated*, either in the same child or in the same family, there is particularly likely to be depression, involving distortion of perspectives. Inappropriate judgement of the situation is imminent and likely to be chronic.

This was, for instance, the case with Kaija, aged six and a half. She was a feeble-minded girl with a cleft palate and cerebral injury acquired during delivery. The parents filled in the inquiry form very sketchily, and both the tone of their answers and the documentation performed in the ward reflected this *contagious* resignation. Medical clarification of the situation remained incomplete in the clinic, even badly so. A similar course of events occurred with nine-year-old Kalle, a feeble-minded, hard-of-hearing, and myopic boy, whose speech was at a very elementary level.

If a defect in an individual, or in a larger unit of society, such as a family, is labelled as a debility, a shortcoming (or even a 'degeneracy'), this is always done on the basis of some communal constellation. Such a constellation is in turn experienced against a background – the image of man and life prevailing in the locality. In modern communities a defect may receive manifold receptions, but one predominant attitude is that of computation. The defect is given an appraisal based on *measurement*. The child is measured according to certain arbitrary norms, which are often regarded as given, and not existing in a context of integration. If the standards are considered self-evident, the child has, as it were, failed to 'measure up', and the threatened potential is now even more threatened: the possibilities are minimal of integrating the potentiality into the individual and the individual into the community. Further distortion of the defect then threatens, and the emergence of destructive processes in the human relations involved. These processes and distortions can still, however, allow one to read – 'hear' – an appeal for integration. But if this appeal too is only received in a computatory spirit, if measurements are made, followed by corrective moves aiming at mere dismissal of the defect from the field, the essence of the appeal is being ignored: the appeal is more seriously threatened and may become mute.

What, for instance, are the possibilities of developmental

integration into the community for a child with damage to the brain (CP)? Clearly the possibilities depend on the community's view. Integration will be much less accessible if it is a predominant axiom in the community that brain injury excludes the victim from normal community life. Again, the more cerebral injury is experienced as a *disconnected* phenomenon, an anonymous accident, a mechanical defect outside the common historical network of human responsibility, the less chance the sufferer has of developmental integration. It would be interesting to know, for instance, whether a progression of the child's cerebral process, or the formation of a destructive scar, might possibly be related to fundamental factors of this kind, but no studies of this sort have been performed.

(b) In the constellations where there is disturbance in speech development, intelligence is of central significance. Speech ability is, in point of fact, a constitutive element and dimension of intelligence. But this does not necessarily imply the capacity for articulated *vocal* speech. Speaking capacity in the widest sense is meant here: any potentiality capable of being developed into a bridge, any talent capable of acting as a vehicle for social communication, will serve. 'Speech' is an encounter in and with symbols; it is comprehending and being comprehensible, giving and receiving comprehension – 'reciprocal comprehensibility' in some 'language'. Employment of a common 'language' is the formation of a shared life worthy of a human being and a human culture. Participating linguistically in his world with others, living in it, every human being becomes, in various ways and degrees, a centre of speech. Here 'intelligence' comes into play: the relative independence, cohesion, integrity, continuity, mobility, and differentiation of this life as a speech centre form dimensions of intelligence.

Talent operates within the framework of reciprocal comprehensibility: within this framework the diversity of talent is considerable. Even if we confine ourselves to purely linguistic talents, there are extremely varied ones. These are only a few: fluency in verbalizing thoughts, feelings, hopes, or demands; articulation of understanding, whether of oneself or of some social unit; verbal evocation of the atmosphere in some intimate or more public circle; verbal expression of various dimensions of the nature surrounding man; verbalization of the tensions and conflicts of interest between people; linguistic evocation of broad historical spans; the recreation of one's own language; the ability to dramatize oneself in a foreign language; skill in discussion or speechmaking; talent for poetry or artistic prose; the articulation of systematic thinking; and so on. If we go on to consider dimensions of reciprocal comprehensibility in general (not confining ourselves to the specifically linguistic), the spectrum is unlimited. Even a short segment suggests the extent of the possibilities, among them: composing music, performing music, pantomime, mathematics, differentiated communication with certain species of animals, comprehension of gesture and social code.

An individual can only guess at a fraction of the potentialities of reciprocal comprehensibility. Even a particular epoch, or one of the diversified communities within a cultural sphere, hardly suspects the wealth available. Certain forms of reciprocal comprehensibility have always been realized, while thousands of other potentialities have either only evolved in fringe areas or have been left completely unexploited. Certain forms of communication acquire dominance, while others are rejected or discouraged. This process of selection and discrimination takes place in various dimensions of reciprocal comprehensibility, in various cultural spheres, within language areas and between them.

This being so, many of our linguistic potentialities may, in fact, be encountered as disturbances of speech-development, or their constellations. The more axiomatic it appears to be that we *already possess* all the necessary reciprocal comprehensibility – that we have it in the normal linguistic practice of what we assume to be a healthy community – the more 'the superfluous', 'the eccentric' will be thrust aside: in this way often very diversified linguistic potentialities and talents are rejected and lost; they are forced into distortion, or suffocated and totally denied admittance. When this happens they may emerge as a peculiarity or a 'defect'.

How does the delusion of having possession – here that we possess all the necessary reciprocal comprehensibility – arise? Nowadays it seems to occur as follows. We conceive of speech as a mere ability or skill and think we know what the standards are – as if they were 'natural', or mechanically given. In this process we are forgetting that speech – in particular – is an integral part of community living and being: that it is inseparable from the community as an organic occurrence, a communal growth, as differentiation and mutual integration.

The less differentiated an individual is in his intelligence, the less able he is, in general, to constitute a centre of speaking capacity. Thus the more he has to speak and understand through others – those who do constitute centres to a greater degree. An oligophrenic is a special example of this. His participation in social communication, language, and speech is peculiarly dependent on the vitality of the community's responsible hierarchy. Not that the 'sparse-minded' person (*oligo* means 'sparse' and not 'defective'!) has nothing to say. It is simply that *disclosure* of what he has to say – and thus his articulated speech – depends with *particular* immediacy on the recognition of his presence. It is thus essential for each oligophrenic's specific quality – and not merely the quality of his defects – to be acknowledged. Even low-frequency vibrations are vibrations, and inalienably part of the common chord.

It was pointed out above that the delusional image of an ideal community contained within it the delusional notion that a normal individual would be capable of autonomous existence in principle. According to this image, the existence of an ordinary 'healthy' human being is fundamentally independent of both his fellow-men and the universe. The following assumption tends to be the starting point: that, for a community to exist properly, all its individuals ought to act as autonomous speaking centres, all more or less equally independent. If one overlooks the organic nature of the community in this manner, one inevitably experiences oligophrenia as definitely and exclusively a mental *deficiency*: the situation is seen as one where a human being – due to some unaccountable caprice of circumstance – has no share in intelligent communication through speech and is permanently sealed off from it. It seems probable that there is projection here: extrusion and location of one's own human 'impoverishment' into the more obvious 'poverty' of this 'sparse-minded' fellow-man, with his meagre intellectual resources. In other words, one cannot allow oneself to experience one's *own* deprivation, one's *own* loss of a sense of community. We do not share our lives: our image of the community has ensured that; and our own experience of ourselves and our life with others is 'sparse', unbearably so. The 'meagreness' must thus be denied, projected, found elsewhere. The more massive such projection is, the greater the latent hopelessness: the more we have despaired about our own resources. We feel that our debt to life is unpayable and therefore unacknowledgeable. Our fear of this unpayable demand on us is associated with our ultimate fear, death, and we are immersed in the projection of our latent death-fear and worship. Oligophrenia is a sitting target for such projection.

A symptom that supports this interpretation is the prevalent modern hypersensitivity to the images that the oligophrenic's appearance, motion, and voice present. The ugliness that the community had dismissed is rearing into view, but now located and visible. Inconspicuously the face of our life together has been prettified out of reality; we have jointly created an idealized picture. When we encounter the visage of meagre intellectual differentiation we feel that we are confronted by ugliness itself, which ought to have been dismissed from the world. This locating process corresponds to the projection of 'stupidity', as reflected for example, in the jokes that the 'intelligent' tell about the mentally retarded. That this confusion of 'stupidity' and meagre intellectual differentiation is typical of the contemporary situation is subtly demonstrated by the German theologian Dietrich Bonhoeffer in his letters (1952) from prison, written during the last war.[1]

The oligophrenic may be 'ill'; that is he does suffer; he behaves embarrassingly, perhaps even destructively; and he speaks defectively, in a disturbing way. But what is this 'illness'? Clearly it

[1] The letters include analyses of 'stupidity'.

is the lack, the non-realization, of communal integration for the patient, or the specific kind he represents. What is the obstacle to integration? It is often precisely the almost exclusive stress on performance and defectiveness in the relations between the patient and his community. Constellations involving some kind of oligophrenia are, to a quite special extent, constructed on communal attitudes, rooted deep in our traditions. Any individual family will thus experience great difficulties in finding a living relation to an oligophrenic member. This is bound to be the case, when the wider community, the greater human family, tends to manifest such meagre participation and responsibility for integration and is dominated by the projections described above.

To what extent are oligophrenics present for us and themselves? In what manner are they present? How far, and in what manner, are oligophrenic features in *ourselves* present to us all? What form does speech take in this situation? The answers to these questions will reveal, in a quite special way, the tension between reality and appearance in the multiple dimensions of speech. The verbal formulations will reveal the tensions and conflicts, the denials and acceptances, inhering in our intercommunication, self-expression, articulation of existing circumstances and expression of existence as a human being.[1]

IV   WHY 'CONSTELLATIONS'?

We have been discussing 'constellations' in the sphere of speech development and its disturbances. Why 'constellations' as a point of departure, and not various well-known and established diagnoses in the field? One reply would be that no undisputedly recognized classification exists. But why constellations? For one thing, the investigational and therapeutic team encountered resistances to diagnosis and therapy that made it impossible to locate the problems at all plausibly in the individual patient, in his symptoms, and syndromes, and confine them there. Nor did the

---

[1] Siirala (1964) includes a historical survey of this tension between integration and splintering, between symbolic and diabolic word formation, in medicine, therapy, philosophy, and theology.

resistances convincingly invite separate treatment. They could not be designated as 'psychic or social factors' and treated in distinction from the supposed 'actual' defect or disease. The afflictions, defects and disease processes themselves provided a resistance, with a configuration organically related to the community's state of integration. The concept of 'the constellation' thus became necessary. It is not offered as a final conceptual solution; rather, it is a way of approach in the pursuit of the most relevant possible encounter with the problems. Clearly, it was chosen because it was considered to open up a more productive line of inquiry than was possible without it. It helped towards an understanding of the nature of the individual organism's defectiveness. Only a preliminary study of the concept will be provided in this chapter. Later chapters will develop the explanation.

The initial clarification will be through examples. Here, in brief outline, are a few illustrations from the phoniatric case records; I shall go on to collate and discuss these.

Reino, aged seven, had a father who was slow in his speech and movements, while the mother was inclined to speak copiously and fast. (She was also myopic.) Immediately after birth the boy had to spend months in an orphanage, due to his parents' tuberculosis. His diagnosis was dyslalia, hypacusis perceptiva, cerebral lesion.

The diagnosis of Paavo, aged seven, was hyperkinesia laryngis. He began to display hoarseness at the age of three. His parents had been in a constant hurry. All four children in the family constantly sucked dummies, including the eldest, who was nine years old.

Esko was nine years old and stuttered. The diagnosis was tachyphemia, dysarthria, dysgraphia, dyslexia, and balbuties. His speech difficulty was very conspicuously dependent on situations. His behaviour was fundamentally hasty throughout. All that could be recovered about his early infancy was that his nest had been to some degree unstable – the child had only been fed irregularly, for example – and that he had also suffered from loss of appetite. The parents thought that the stuttering began when Esko ran way from home at the age of five and was spanked for it.

Then there was Leila, aged seven and a half, who had difficulties in reading and writing, as well as a speech disturbance, which was something between stuttering and cluttering. In addition, there was agrammatism. The girl's physical growth was exceptionally slow until the age of five; but later she made up the difference. (She learned to walk, however, at a standard age, thirteen months.) When Leila was four years old she accidentally bit her tongue, which was sutured and healed well. In the ward the girl proved rather more infantile than other children of the same age, and her intelligence was calculated as on the borderline between normal and poorly endowed. Leila had a poor vocabulary, her sentences were clumsy, and long words caused difficulties in articulation. On the other hand she was capable of rather complex communication. For instance, she organized singing games in the ward with other children, inventing words for the songs herself. As to the family, it was established that the girl's mother and brother learned to speak late, and that the mother suffered from migraine. The questionnaire completed by the mother indicated that the father of the family 'bothers and teases children'.

Heikki, with the echo-speech, described in detail above, will be included with this group. It will then be possible to perform comparisons, seek common factors and make distinctions. It is, for instance, possible to categorize the patients on the basis of those with obvious suggestions of cerebral defect or damage, and those without such indications. A further category would be the patients with disturbance of speech development in the family. An obvious basis for classification would also be speech disturbances as distinct from vocal disturbances. Syndrome diagnosis is also possible: Esko's and Leila's difficulties can be identified as tachyphemia, etc.

I think a productive line of inquiry, however, would be from the angle of *hurry* in speech: that is, the sense of insufficient human time for reciprocal comprehension, or at least for certain essential situations in which it might be cultured. For Reino the conflicting speech images provided by the parents presented a problem: the mother's hasty delivery and the father's extreme slowness. Possibly this implied the transmission of a particular gene combination from the parents to their child; however that may be, a certain chronic disturbance of rhythm had certainly been created in the speech milieu of the nest. As regards the time dimension of the nest itself, Reino missed out on several initial months. How radical the deficiency was could not be recollected. But, since Spitz's studies, it is common knowledge that several months' separation from the mother during early infancy is a serious threat to the child's development; the severity depends on how capable the substitute environment is of fulfilling an individual maternal function for the child.

Paavo's parents too were in a constant hurry – and the boy himself had developed laryngeal hyperkinesia, a designation that speaks for itself. That all the children in the family were constantly hungry for the dummy would suggest that the parents' hurry had led to some primary need being overlooked.

All Esko's behaviour was hurried, including his speech. Leila, again, had developed different speeds: both a normal rapidity and an extreme slowness. She had had a classic hasty accident, injuring her tongue with her teeth!

And then Heikki: his parents' time was reserved for elsewhere, away from the child; it was consumed in convulsive monomania, the pursuit of a 'higher standard of living', and in seeking the mother-in-law's good opinion (as a representative of other people). There was latent despair. Heikki's mother even felt she was 'neglecting her work' if she took time off for her son. Hurry was thus supported by 'conscience'; with such moral authority, hurry would have the force to influence the elementary preconditions for Heikki's speech. Hurry was a structural element in the boy's tendency towards autistic behaviour. This became clearly apparent from his reaction to the opposite of hurry: if a ward lady hummed in Heikki's vicinity, the boy would stop his tantrum immediately and try to climb into the lady's lap. In the vocal dimension, humming is specifically a manifestation of un-hurriedness: it is disengaged, unpurposeful: there is no sense of time pressing, or an urgent future.

Hurry in speech implies the child's sense that there is insufficient time available for the recognition and acceptance of his presence. The child feels that there is not enough time to express himself and be heard. In my view this quality of hurry is centrally characteristic of all the constellations described above. I don't claim, of course, that the hurried speech constellation in any way excludes other diagnostic characterizations, performed from other points of view. I argue that it *is* inadequate to interpret cases of disturbed speech *solely* as structural faults, defects in performance by individual organisms, and the combination of these in syn-dromes. I claim that it is not enough if these diagnoses are subse-quently connected with 'psychic', 'social', and 'environmental' factors: the shortcoming of this approach is that the disease con-figuration does not encounter us thus. The configuration that encounters us when the responsibility has not been primarily the-matized is that of a compact unity: the facts are structured into a constellation. Even primarily, the individual organism's structural faults and defects in performance are revealed as constituent features of the individual's deficiency of reciprocal communal integration. The problem and challenge this poses meets us from the first. This applies to illness in general, although speech dis-turbances perhaps manifest the fact with particular potency.

The confrontation with constellations implies, as has already become apparent, some accounting with certain customary habits of thought. An analysis follows of two constellations in which patients were deafened, and one hardness-of-hearing constella-tion. I studied the first two for extended periods in the consulta-tions. I read the third as a case history. The analysis, however, demands preliminary clarification of concepts. Both speaking and listening are integral parts of reciprocal comprehension. Both articulated speech and audition with hearing organs inherently belong to speaking and listening, yet neither is indispensable. Speech or hearing in the widest sense of these conceptions can proceed without vocal speech or the hearing organs. Speech can be transposed into writing or tactile signals; hearing can be replaced by lip-reading or the deciphering of tactile signals; and so on.

Speech and hearing, in fact, like various other aspects of human existence, cannot be unambiguously localized, exhaustively defined, or even characterized with the traditional objectification. Nevertheless, both speech and hearing – in the narrower senses – can be objectified in the most diversified ways; and this makes possible even more complex influences on the realization of the ability to speak and hear.

Hearing can be regarded, for instance, as a series of events constructed on the basis of the most diversified preconditions, involving modifications of forms of energy and systems of signals. In ordinary existence such auditory facts are not in the foreground, although they form the constant structural details of hearing. But they are by no means the sole structural details or dimensions of hearing; nor are they the only ones that are concealed from us. As a function, hearing is more unambiguously localized than is articulated speech; and yet hearing too *is* man's being: it is man who hears, and not the middle ear, or Cort's organ, or the cerebral cortex, although they do participate in hearing.

As for speech, the fundamental prerequisites for hearing do not live a separate life in any organ or part of an organ. In order to develop, articulated speech requires acceptance of the speaker's presence. Hearing, again, presupposes that what is presented for hearing *can* be heard in a *human* sense: a child, for instance, cannot tolerate hearing anything that is in immediate conflict with the fundamental factors of his total security. The child can certainly tolerate hearing a danger signal; but a child will not readily hear, for instance, that he will only be acceptable to his parents if he goes on performing something that is actually impossible for him.

Raimo, for instance, was admitted to the phoniatric ward. Even at the age of four he had been forced to look after his baby brother all day long; this even involved ensuring that the six-month-old baby was put on his chamber-pot. The purpose was to free his parents for their other interests. Raimo could readily be directed through auditory channels: he was compliant in the most radical sense of the word. But at some stage he started to 'neglect' his duties, was then impetuously blamed by his parents, and the boy became partially deaf. In the ward Raimo at first behaved very obediently, but after a couple of weeks a most disobedient boy emerged. The point was that here it was possible for his own will, for which there was scarcely any room at home, to emerge in childish defiance.

Aino, again, an eleven-year-old girl, stopped hearing, although no organic defect in her auditory organs was detectable on examination. Her deafness, gradually revealed to be selective, had indeed been preceded by dizziness – which is traditionally regarded as an 'organic' symptom. In the course of the child's individual psychotherapy with the team's psychologist and meetings between the mother and the team's social worker, the following picture emerged. Aino's parents had a 'forced' marriage, due to extramarital pregnancy. Thus the responsibility for acceptance of the role of spouse and parent had largely devolved on to circumstance and an impropriety. Aino's mother had been too shy to take up and disentangle conflicts with the husband, though only the sketchiest picture of the husband's point of view on this could be obtained. Even as a very little child Aino had been bothered by assorted fears. She was unable to develop any kind of observable emotional response to the birth of her younger brother – but was driven to enuresis in this connection. (Aino was extremely afraid of travel by water: she vomited even before a boat trip.) The girl developed an especially conspicuous dependence on her mother. In the ward she manifested a peculiar combination of erotically-toned stimulation and simultaneous rejection of sexuality. About a year before she became deaf, Aino suffered from insomnia, ate meagrely, and deteriorated in her school performance. On the night of the first of May (an occasion of celebration in Finland) she happened to hear her parents having sexual intercourse, and she became deaf. In the course of several months' psychotherapy and other therapeutic relationships in the ward she gradually managed to relinquish her selective non-hearing – though remnants persisted. Taken as a whole, Aino's case shows features of nervous anorexia; deafness, however, dominates the picture, and it led to early treatment, perhaps before the nervous anorexia had time to develop completely.

Aino's deafness had quite clearly been developed as an elementary protection against what she was incapable of accepting. The unacceptable, sexuality, was specifically associated with the stage of puberty: this was developing exceptionally early: menstruation was in sight, and the signs of pubescence were visible in many of her class-mates. The family was offering Aino very little support towards acceptance of her role of woman. As a matter of fact, what she heard at home would discourage the woman in her. Her mother – the representative of womanhood and maternity on her horizon – was ill equipped to defend her role or position: in fact she had 'nothing to say' in this area. The parents' experience of each other as sexual beings was conducted in an atmosphere of conflict and confusion, and there was no verbal expression of its feebleness and the associated tensions. Thus, when Aino happened to overhear sexual communication taking place between man and woman, she could not cope with the experience: there was no even incipiently organized and secure framework into which she could accommodate the encounter.

If a congenitally hard-of-hearing child can find no other means of defending his being, he may resort to his hearing difficulty for defence. Also, a defect may become a child's principal means of obtaining what he wants.

A relevant instance is Riitta, who was in the ward when she was two, and again between the ages of five and six. Her left external ear had been deformed, and the auditory canal on that side had had to be opened surgically. The girl still heard very poorly at the age of six and could only speak one word-symbol; however, she could express herself skilfully by means of sign language, accompanying her gestures with energetic vociferation. The child was shy, suspicious, and inclined to withdraw into hearing defectiveness, and, on the other hand, willing for contact, active and co-operative in certain respects. She was clearly intelligent too. The central question was why the child had to resort to her defective hearing. But the parents lived in a remote district and could not be brought effectively into investigation of the situation and the child's treatment, and thus the question remained unclarified. Also, the more precise nature of the hearing defect remained obscure as regards both organ function and Riitta's poor static co-ordination.

The comprehensive picture, therefore, never became more than superficial, although clarification was urgently needed for the child's development.

The hearing impairment patterns of Raimo, Aino, and Riitta were rather different. Only in the case of Riitta did backwardness in articulated speech constitute an actual and central problem. For Raimo and Aino the direct emphasis was on how to endure hearing, how to undertake the task of digesting the words spoken to them. On this particular point, Riitta had already arrived at another stage; she was settled in her hearing defect. For all three, however, the conflict – about whether to participate in reciprocal social comprehension or withdraw – was still unresolved, still in progress. But in different ways the conflict had been canalized as the onset of a hearing disorder; and the reifiable and objectifiable bodily dimension – or, to use the traditional term, the 'organic' dimension – had been affected in varying degrees.

In the case of Aino, it soon became apparent to the team that there was a correlation between the actual hearing ability and the problem of tolerance. Even the girl's parents had some inkling of the matter. They consequently agreed to accept the prolonged psychotherapy suggested for Aino, although they did so very ambivalently and interrupted the therapy from time to time.

In the case of Raimo, the responsibility for the family's constellation had already been placed on the boy's hearing defect. The defect did not, however, reveal the direct and continuous relationship to tolerance that was so evident in the case of Aino. On the other hand, the onset of the hearing impairment was still recent enough; and so, in their meetings with the child and his parents, the social worker and the psychologist were able to identify the central factors in the pattern of impaired hearing that the family's constellation showed. Here, however, pressure was encountered from the traditional medical attitude. Since indisputable organic fault could be detected, it was indicated that the therapeutic staff had no moral right to be implicated in more than the direct, immediate, and manipulatory treatment of the defect. The boy's development, and possibly the future of his hearing too, made prolonged and thorough treatment of his family constellation essential. Yet there was no provision for this within the tradition. Thus the possibility of involving the parents in personally responsible co-operation could not even be given a trial.

In the case of Riitta no such possibility even emerged. There were too many obstacles, starting with the remoteness of the family home. And whereas the origin of Raimo's hearing impairment was still recent history, the pattern of Riitta's impairment had become stabilized. The pressure of medical tradition was even more categorical in the case of Riitta: it would be neither valuable nor permissible to spend public funds and resources on clarifying the total situation and activating the child's native community to accept its share of responsibility for the disease constellation.

Thus the most multiple dimensions are involved. Dimensions actually quite remote from the patient's organism – in this case medical authority – and his family relations are operative in deciding the extent to which an impediment in the communal speaking and hearing situation becomes the permanent responsibility of an individual's organs.

As pointed out before, all human sense-experience, including hearing, is *human*: man's sense experience is part of his humanity, part of his human being as a human entity. The 'results' we

obtain in measuring organic functions are not the mere performances of organs: they are also invariably – and this includes,
for instance, the EEG tracings in a medical examination of
hearing – the performances of a man: we are witnessing global
human behaviour in the organ. The organ, and even the cell, do
behave within the organism and from the organism, although they
are not centres of behaviour in the sense that the man himself is.

If an organ or cell starts behaving autonomously, this implies
illness or incipient illness. There is no basis for such autonomy:
it is against the natural prerequisites of an organ or tissue. The
most drastic form of quasi-autonomy is malignancy: the hubristic
growth of cell tissue, regardless of the rest of the organism. In
general the behaviour of an organ can be integrated in the existence of the total organism in various ways and degrees. But just
as the behaviour of an individual who is unintegrated into his
community becomes in some respect disorganized and distorted,
so it is with an organ that is defectively integrated into the total
organism.

This would scarcely be denied by anyone, as an analogy. However, it is not generally accepted, or even recognized, that there
is a connection between the individual's integration into the community and the organ's integration into the organism. Indeed,
the existence of such an association is difficult to demonstrate
verifiably in terms of reductive reification, or objectified knowledge for the sake of control.[1] Since I want to develop the point
that there is a connection between the individual's communal
integration and the integration of organs in the organism, it may
help if I first present a schematic view of the relation.

Apparently, a pattern of events such as the following may
occur. There is some disintegration – which I call an historic
constellation: some failure has intruded between the community
and the individual. This failure to integrate is one that cannot
penetrate into awareness, into communal, responsible consciousness: it prevails as a latent communal crisis. Certain types of

---

[1] Primary control, as complete as possible, of all that encounters man as sickness
seems to represent the governing trend in medicine, at least implicitly; the attain-
ment of generally valid knowledge through objectification and reduction.

individual are particularly vulnerable to this crisis: for them the crisis becomes crucial: the dilemma in the whole constellation is transferred to them, becomes the burden of such an individual. Perhaps this person who has been made solely responsible will be able to develop a crisis now at a semi-communal, semi-personal level: a neurosis, let us say, or, at the price of the destruction of his social entity, a psychosis. Such crises are indirect appeals to the community. But physical illness too is, in a certain sense, a way of expressing the dilemma – but a more concealed, muffled, and inarticulate alarm.[1]

In *physical* illness the community's failure in integration has even bypassed individual personality: it has become the burden of an anonymous organ. The organ, or organ system, which is intrinsically concerned in the situation – such as Raimo's auditory organs, which transmitted the demand for unlimited obedience – breaks down and manifests illness when it has to bear the full responsibility in isolation. Such inappropriate delegation of responsibility occurs when the problem is unintegrated into the community: both the community and the individual evade consciousness and responsibility, and the responsibility passes on out of the human sphere. The organ's fulfilment of its specific ability becomes difficult or even impossible under such circumstances: it has been given a responsibility that is not only unamenable but beyond its capacity. It cannot bear it alone and breaks under the burden. Such vicarious illness – the organ suffering for the whole organism, and the individual suffering for the community – is, many researchers now believe, one of the basic dimensions of being ill.

A later analysis in this study is designed to show that such vicariousness is the basic channel in the causal process of disease.

[1] Viktor von Weizsäcker, the German internist and neurologist who died in 1956, and several of his pupils have systematically illustrated this process with supporting clinical examples and have analysed it in numerous books and articles. Psychosomatic medicine, based on traditional psychoanalysis, has implicitly arrived at similar conclusions, although not, for the most part, in such general human terms.

CHAPTER 3

Aetiology

I CONTROL THROUGH REDUCTION: THE DOMINANT ATTITUDE IN MEDICINE

The concept of cause is employed in medicine in many widely differing forms. The implications of this are rarely clarified. We talk for instance of a disease picture, a syndrome, a clinical picture, or the like. Then, in the course of our investigation, we conclude that such and such a disease process or agent has emerged as the cause. The disease we have discovered here constitutes the producer of the symptoms: it is a sort of 'formal cause', the *causa formalis* of antiquity. The more primary agent, on the other hand, corresponds to part of the 'efficient cause', the *causa efficiens* of antiquity. These two usages of the concept 'cause' are probably differentiated in principle, however, even when the difference is not expressed in words. But in the traditional use of the concept of 'cause' there are other kinds of implicit attitudes, and these are of a much more fundamentally problematic character.

Medical thinkers are, it is true, aware of disorientations, even numerous ones, that are characteristic of current causal thinking. There is the *post hoc-propter hoc* deduction; or there are attempts to explain a speech disturbance on the basis of a single causative factor; there is contentment with the disclosure of a short causal chain in a situation where explication should be pursued further; there is the tendency to use some generally recognized causative factor as a 'scapegoat', as a location for all the difficulties encountered in examination and therapy; and there is disregard of the so-called 'psychic' factors. Important as such observations concerning medical attitudes are, their prophylactic or corrective effect upon errors does not, I think, penetrate deeply enough into the foundations of the disorientating attitudes. The nature of one's most axiomatic, and as such often completely legitimate-seeming, conceptions needs to be analysed within a broader human perspective. This perspective – or rather a background screen on to which the projection has to take place – is not and cannot be included in any current scientific medical system itself, as its 'technical element'.

One possibility in this direction is to ask: what is the quality and being of the particular disease process or agent that is regarded as the cause? Whatever else it may be, it is the following in the mainstream of medicine, at least: a characteristically repeated phenomenal whole, expressed and approached through the concepts of natural science: concepts, that is, in the service of a reductive, universally applicable control. But in that case what is the quality (essence) and being of the concepts of natural science themselves – these instruments of 'grasping', of *Begriffe*? It is too easily forgotten that these very concepts, whereby one 'grasps' and conceives the cause or 'producer' of the disease phenomenon, have themselves been 'produced' in our processes of perception. They have originated in the perceptive processes in the course of the pursuit of reductive controlling knowledge. They are thus elements of a certain style of approach and action, a style selected from innumerable other possibilities. Nevertheless, they are by no means subject to chance; there is no question of that, of course. On the contrary, within the limits of their own laws and their areas of application, it is rather unambiguously possible to detect what is 'valid' and what is not. They efficiently serve the pursuit of generally valid control. But on the other hand they do not reveal the 'ultimate reality' of anything except their own 'validity'. In spite of their assistance we have not 'grasped', even in principle, the 'ultimate reality' of the phenomena.

It is odd, and also significant, that although doctors are aware of this, in principle, to some degree, there is nevertheless still an opposite tendency in medicine. The disease processes, as figured in natural scientific terms, tend to be regarded as the 'ultimate' underlying causal influences and sources 'behind' things that are actually encountered in other terms. This is even true, in principle, of the depth psychology working on the natural scientific model. In the physiology of the senses, too, in the research on the event of perception itself, a similar basic approach has tended to dominate. Indeed, this research has been pursuing 'causes' for the perceptions that the test subject reports (about the 'exterior world' or the 'interior world' of the body) in the stimuli and/or in the transmission processes within the body. Reenpää (1962) has demonstrated the problematic character of this mode of thinking, which assumes that there is a causal chain proceeding from a stimulus and a stimulation process into perception. He has, in fact, succeeded in analysing how the precise natural scientific concepts employed for describing stimuli and stimulation processes are themselves constructed, in quite definite and specific ways, out of our – quantitatively – elementary sensory experiences.

Viktor von Weizsäcker (1940) showed the mutual inter-involvement of an investigator's perception and movement (including mental movement) and analysed the significance for physiological research. He and his school – in particular Wilhelm Kütemeyer – subsequently performed relevant case history studies and analyses of doctor-patient relationships for the internal medical patients in their care. In this way they were able to clarify the position of the investigator in relation to his object of medical study. When sick patients were treated in terms of von Weizsäcker's 'anthropological medicine', the image that had dominated human investigators for centuries – that of an observer having a position independent of his object of study, the observed – was found unsatisfactory. This image was systematically shown to conflict irresolvably with the experience of disease as an event. A huge body of similar evidence already exists through Freud's psychoanalysis and Freudian psychotherapeutic treatment and research.[1] Inspired by Freud, and working directly with the world of experience of bodily illness, von Weizsäcker saw more

[1] Systematic conclusions from this have, however, rarely been drawn within psychoanalytic circles proper.

clearly than others the central role that this misconception of an 'independent observer' was playing; he saw that medical research was impoverished by it, and that the error played a part in the origin and maintenance of disease.

The concept of an independent observer, or a primarily autonomous position, is deeply rooted in human history. The course of the concept in the West has been analysed by many contemporary philosophers, theologians, and writers, and, more rarely, by medical scientists.[1] We will only point out here that the species of objectifying controlling knowledge known as 'natural science' is not the first position man has adopted under the misconception – delusion, even – of possessing a completely independent starting-point or primary autonomy. In other words, the natural-scientific tradition has merely replaced an earlier reductive reification, or delusion of achieved knowledge, associated with explicitly religious symbols. The question thus concerns a position that man imagines (more properly, assumes – for conscious imaging does not come into it) he possesses: a position of self-sufficiency, free from fundamental dependency. According to this delusion, man is the origin of all – at least of all understanding – and thus himself determines his own basic responsibility. In this condition man also implicitly assumes that he has not become involved in any obscuring and distorting delusion, at least in essentials.

It is insufficient here to recognize the relativity, the 'human error factor', in reductive controlling knowledge. It is also essential to seek the natural place of each mode of investigation and encounter (including the precise objectification of 'natural science') within the whole, within the manifold hierarchical order of modes of encounters. The theory of relativity is one impressive example of utilizing insight into the relativity of man's observation, within a specific system of reductive controlling knowledge. And although Reenpää's and von Weizsäacker's analyses, for instance, relativize the traditional modes of operating

[1] The significance of this particular delusional position for the schizophrenia situation (including the patient, the society surrounding him, the disease process and our attitude towards it) is described in my *Die Schizophrenie – des Einzelnen und der Allgemeinheit* (Schizophrenia in the Individual and the Community).

with the concept of cause in medicine, this is not, of course, to say that the existing information concerning causes has been proved invalid. On the contrary, the possibility is now beginning to take form of seeing reductive controlling knowledge in its own place within the whole perspective: its special nature can be progressively recognized in a more nuanced way. In principle, the potentialities of that control know no limits. On the other hand, limitations are often inherent in the delusion of being in an axiomatically given and 'absolutely real' mode of encountering disease.

In the case of disturbed speech development, the disease is inevitably encountered in such manifold ways, including ones where we ourselves are involved, that an exclusive, primary (and not even conscious) aspiration for reductive control makes us overlook the most essential aspects. These aspects, these challenges for research, are often essential for precisely the aspiration towards reductive control. If, however, the causal information obtained through the endeavour is allowed to pass for a total answer to the causal problem in a disease constellation, we shall be misled. Reduction always identifies the cause for the sake of certain limited information, measures, and control: it does not represent more than a quite specific aspect of the causal network and our relation to it.

II THE PRIMACY OF THE REDUCTIVE ATTITUDE, AND ITS INFLUENCE ON INTERPRETATION AND TREATMENT

It often seems as if investigators regarded the concepts and problem setting of traditional reductive control as constituting a totally isolated area; as if, even in principle, there could be no point of contact – at least no scientific point of contact – with the shared world of common sense and other insights into vital connections, however pertinent. Landau *et al.* (1960) reported a case of aphasia in a child, a scoliotic and mildly diplegic boy with a congenital heart condition (Taussig–Bing). Through prolonged and particularly devoted special training, the child achieved a considerable mastery of speech. The autopsy finding, when the boy suddenly died in connection with mumps, was consequently a considerable surprise for the investigators: the primary auditory thalamocortical projectory system, without which speech is considered impossible, was destroyed in the boy's brain. (There were old infarctions in the region of the Sylvian fissures and retrograde degeneration in the nuclei of the medial geniculate body.) The writers concluded that the auditory understanding function of the child must have employed other brain tracts than those customarily regarded as absolutely specific for these functions. This observation is undoubtedly important, and the conclusion clear. But many questions spring to mind and these are ultimately involved with the problem Landau and his associates have dealt with.

The occurrence reported in the article is, it would seem, significant enough in nature to deserve a more differentiated investigation. This case seems to present a breakthrough comparable to the case of Anne Sullivan and Helen Keller, which involved blindness and deafness. The reciprocal comprehension with the boy proceeded from a most elementary level: the six-year-old boy did not comprehend articulated speech, and only through helpless gestures and sounds was it clear that he wished to convey a meaning. Yet speaking communication was eventually achieved. In the St Louis Institute for the Deaf, then, a persistently responsible and devoted reception was available for the boy and his dilemma and proved sufficient to enable the child to mobilize successfully his remaining (speech-communication) resources.

It must again be emphasized that speech is never merely an objective occurrence: it is never realized merely locally, or in an individual. Speech, in fact, also occurs as a communication *between* human beings; it is a structural mode of a supra-individual reality. It reveals quite specifically that man always is, always exists, outside himself as well as within himself: that the being of man has a mode of 'ex-sistence', of standing outside. This will be more fully dealt with in the following chapter. Of course, in speech many objectively observable factors occur *also*, both in the individual and his environment; but the 'also' is crucial.

At the age of ten the boy suddenly died 'in connection with' mumps. To quote the authors, this was 'probably because of a cardiac complication'.[1] The word 'probably' in this context implies that the result of the autopsy did not provide indisputable information. If we now survey the boy's phases as a whole, such an explanation of his death surely proves unsatisfactory. Here, in fact, it was not merely a blood-pump or a central nervous system that died, but a human being. And a human being's death is always in some way bound up with what precisely, in fact, he is: his death is an event in the history of his specific being and unique course of life. In addition, then, the death of an individual is always the distinctive history of a dimension of life that this individual represented in the community. In what way the death of an individual constitutes waste and destruction, and how far, is not decided solely on the basis of the concrete particulars of the symptoms. Another decisive factor is the nature of the process going on between human beings, the death of the boy being an event and a stage in the relations with other people. The death of this boy, the death of a speech 'prodigy', raises many relevant questions. What changes were occurring at the time in his crucial constellations? Had the boy by any chance lost the closest of his teachers? Had anything special occurred in his family situation? Perhaps there is a more specific question. Had his amazing success in learning to speak somehow led to a constellation where progressive success on this front seemed to have become the basis of his acceptability to other people in general?

Perhaps, in connection with the parotitis, the boy was also suffering from mild encephalitis? If so, he might have been experiencing how fragile the bodily framework was in which his speaking capacity – his card of admittance to existence – rested. Even otherwise, his speech ability would almost certainly have made him sensitively aware of its dependence on other immediate

[1] The medical linguistic formulas continue with astonishing persistence, even where experience has demonstrated the untenableness of the notion corresponding to the formula. The concept 'cause of death' is in question here. It is obvious, is it not, that no isolated factor constitutes the cause of death? The crucial issue is always the individual's pathway to death and his *manner* of dying. The customary use of language here is misleading and distorts the scientific approaches.

prerequisites – such as other people's special willingness to listen, their patience, and their preparedness to understand. In this respect the boy's situation was very much like that of a child during its first year of life, structurally – for then only the mother properly understands her child's verbal and other communications. There was, however, a significant difference. Since the boy was now 'cured', he would be regarded as able to speak. This performance might – almost as the price of the great therapeutic investment in him – be particularly expected of him. Perhaps too the ten-year-old was being approached by specific challenges to incorporate himself into a wider community on a speech basis: perhaps some new stage of school was on the horizon; or perhaps some change in the family conditions was now confronting him with new demands on the speech front. It is conceivable that only the boy fully surmised the dependence of his speech capacity on the readiness of his environment to understand and support him. Perhaps, too, he alone understood its dependence upon the familiarity of the environment. Even the institute's therapeutic team may have been insufficiently aware that the mutual speech integration achieved was so uniquely delicate that an interchange of such rare vitality, a communal intercommunication of the same order, could hardly be anticipated in the wider community, in the world at large. If the coming situation loomed as an impossible cul-de-sac for the boy, little other escape from the dilemma would offer itself but death, which, as it happened, was always in a sense available because of his heart condition. Learning to speak, it must be remembered, was the boy's key to a meaningful part in the shared life. Some feature in the constellation surrounding the child may now have supported the despairing assumption that the continuance of his share in the communal life was absolutely bound up with his still threatened ability to perform. If so, where could he look within this framework if he wanted to find the likelihood of an endurable extension of his life? For we do know that this scale of investment in speech performance is precisely disposed to handicap the very performance, which has been achieved with such effort.

Clearly, in relation to this particular boy, my train of thought has had to be speculative to a degree. The point is this, however: the discussion may perhaps reveal the limitations that are imposed on the scientific pursuit of truth if the problems are confined within narrowly conceived cause-and-effect thinking and the customary terminology. Too many questions are unasked. In this case the point of departure is a remarkable observation concerning a child: the cerebral tracts traditionally considered necessary prerequisites for hearing and understanding had been destroyed, and yet the child had learned to speak. But how had this plasticity of the individual and the community come about? How had speech communication come into being despite such a radical defect? These are surely relevant questions. Yet the only answer available in the article is that there must, then, be other cerebral tracts available for speech. Inevitably, therefore, another area of diagnostic problems and other potentialities for research have been neglected: the possible ultimate connections between the boy's speech condition and his sudden death have remained unexplored. Speech has been dealt with as if it were an individual word-production unit, and not a dimension and constructor of human life and human society.[1]

III BASIC FORMS OF CAUSE-DETECTION; VARIOUS FORMS OF KNOWLEDGE AND CORRESPONDING RESPONSIBILITIES

Not only are there multifarious causes for disease constellations – and health constellations, be it noted – but the pathways along which the search for a cause must necessarily move are also extremely varied. The pursuit of cause always occurs from a particular angle, and there can only be pursuit of particular causes: 'cause in general' is an impossibility even as a conception. Varying according to the nature of each particular situation, the search for cause has, for instance, a time-reference: the area of search is localized to the current time, or to the immediate past,

---

[1] Clearly there is no reason to criticize the approach of these particular authors nor any point; the article here only serves as an example of one prevailing trend in contemporary medicine.

or in some cases, even to the more distant past. In other words, a configuration with a certain time-dimension is aimed at. The cause may at times also be appropriately looked for in the future, in the sense that some new configuration – a disease constellation, for example – may be in process; the future phenomenon must be visualized as a whole, to some extent, if the quality of the cause is to be comprehended to a meaningful degree. We cannot escape from the influence that the *framework* of our search for causes imposes upon our approach to the problems: it is impossible for anyone. But what we can do and clearly 'ought to do' is to be as responsibly aware as possible of *what* we are doing and of the relation our procedure has to the framework of the disease situation that challenges us. Our equipment is at its most feeble if we neither recognize nor acknowledge any dependence or relativity.

Another handicap is not to realize that one is using the concept of cause with quite different meanings in different contexts. For example, textbooks (cf. Sonninen, 1964, p. 53) may variously allege hearing impairments, mental retardation, emotional disorders, and aphasia, with its various sub-forms, as causes of delayed speech development. In that case we have a sample of the parallel usage of quite unparallel causal concepts. When aphasia is proposed as the cause of delayed speech development, the actual meaning is (for instance) this: the syndrome designated aphasia – a disputed and most divergently understood one, by the way, especially where children are concerned – is one of the forms of delayed speech development. Again, where mental deficiency is adduced, the expression means that delayed speech development is often a component of low-grade intellectual differentiation. A third meaning is involved when hearing impediments are indicated as causes: that the inability to hear vocal or articulated speech, or difficulty in doing so, also makes the learning of articulated speech difficult. The expression 'emotional disturbances', on the other hand, constitutes a conglomeration of 'causes': virtually all the other dimensions of man's being are simultaneously being referred to, and it is difficult to grasp what could be conveyed by such a massive announcement, asserting that all these many dimensions are one possible cause. Some aspect of an individual patient's situation may, of course, be slightly illuminated by indicating that such and such a person can immediately recognize the lability of this particular patient's emotional reactions. But beyond this the significance of the statement hardly extends.

Different circumstances also operate as causes in quite different ways. The temporal and local modes of influence, for instance, differ from each other decisively. One need only think, say, of a hereditary constellation as opposed to damage to the genotype: these are very different in their causative nature. Or there is Rh-incompatibility compared with deafness originating in conjunction with meningitis. There is birth trauma as opposed to rejection, or even abandonment, by the parents. This is leaving out of account such matters as the realization of a communal image in the mode of life of a society, with the consequent types of discrimination. And what about the causes operative in various forms of neglect: neglect as the exclusion of some basic and essential human need from consideration, or neglect in the form of not making some necessary existential decision?

The search for a cause may, of course, be primarily limited in many ways. The sphere of search may be limited so as not to encompass any problems except those that can be (at least apparently) controlled manipulatorily. Or one can make a preliminarily unlimited search for causes in principle, but subsequently, in dealing with the findings, divide the causes into the 'scientific' and the 'non-scientific', classifying as scientific the causes that are verifiable through reductive controlling methods. The unsatisfactoriness of the latter procedure is obvious, however, from the state of the traditional forms of reductive controlling science – natural science, that is – itself. If all the medical knowledge that would not stand up to a demand for experimental verification were eliminated, the remaining medicine would be slender indeed. And even the information that does prove verifiable is unmanageably diversified, not at all uniform in nature. Within the scope of natural science the most multidimensional observations are made – and thus correspondingly multfarious 'causes' too are encountered. An illusion of uniformity of knowledge can, however, be maintained by effectively isolating the group of concepts associated with the study. In this way the multidimensionality and ambiguity of a process can remain undetected through the narrowness of the scope imposed.

There are weighty grounds for making a clear distinction between confirmed and unconfirmed knowledge: to avoid, for instance, being led into disorientating subjectivism. Without such a distinction, the systematic accumulation of knowledge is very difficult, if not totally impossible. Distinguishing between tested knowledge and assumption is an indication of respect for the dignity of the object of study, as well as being an acknowledgement of the scientist's fundamental task. Verification, however, only 'loses' its ambiguity when the reductive controlling method of encountering man and his illness is applied in isolation. In an actual encounter with a disease constellation reductive control necessarily represents only one side of the situation existing between the patient and those who are treating him. The verifiability of the knowledge in no way guarantees that the control involved will find its correct place within the factual whole. The verifiable knowledge always contains its own temptation to be understood as an answer to questions it does not in fact answer. In addition, the 'knowledge' may lead to the extinction of problem-setting that would be essential from the point of view of the total situation. As suggested previously, the question of cause arises in many organically different forms and on different levels. The differences are characterized by, among other things, different degrees of reducibility and different degrees of controllability.

In its purest forms the knowledge obtained by the methods of reductive control serves two purposes: it provides a tool for controlling the situation through the dismissal of the offending symptoms – through, for instance, vaccination, an operation, or the use of antibiotics; or it reveals the unchangeable aspect of the constellation – a cerebral tissue defect, or an hereditary disturbance of the metabolism, perhaps.

It has been possible to show statistically that early separation from the mother leads to disturbances in both the bodily, the intellectual, and the character development. The conceptual characterization and circumscription of this vitally important 'motherhood' is, however, by no means without its ambiguities; in fact, if an attempt is made to apply in reductive controlling practice the confirmed knowledge concerning separation from the mother, one encounters the most involved problems. These include the communal attitude towards illegitimate motherhood, prevailing concepts about the essence of a baby, concepts concerning the essentials for the care and education of an infant, the jurisdictional practices of the society, etc.

And then there are such dimensions of knowledge as 'dynamic' or, more specifically, psychoanalytic psychology. A large section of the researchers considered as belonging to this discipline regard their branch of science as biological, and, as such, an area of natural scientific reductive control. Nevertheless, verification or statistical proof has not even been attempted for more than a small fraction of the elements that combine to form its system of knowledge. It seems likely, too, that such confirmation would only be possible to a limited extent and for a small part of the area of research and knowledge. The dilemma might seem resolvable by excluding this species of cognizance from the body of professionally valid knowledge. But against this is the fact that our attitude towards our patients and their diseases always contains some implicit, and possibly unconscious, interpretation of the dynamic of the patient's behaviour – dynamics in the most varied dimensions. The present study's position on the matter is clear: it attempts to show how, in encounters with disease, the doctor's (and other medical personnel's) implicit interpretations come into play in the most varied dimensions: dimensions by no means confined to those in which traditional natural scientific medicine operates, even as extended by the postulates of psychoanalysis or dynamic psychology.

Voluntarily or not, one inevitably has particular conceptions of disease, of which one is usually scarcely conscious, possibly not realizing that another relevant approach to the problem even exists. The implicit conceptions cannot, however, be eliminated by establishing that they lie outside the field of reductive controlling knowledge. We are forced to take a stand towards our conceptions and take responsibility for them – and for the stand as well. It is difficult for this assumption of responsibility to become capable of application and fertile, if our actions are dominated by the illusion of moving in one dimension of knowledge only. Again, if questions arise organically in connection with the examination and treatment of patients, would it not be untoward to push the questions aside because no ready labels are available or because one cannot see in advance how far and in what sense the insight and knowledge they offer can be verified?

A relevant instance of such potential knowledge is the anthropological analysis of speech presented in this study. This seems to provide the possibility for the development of a specific type of observational research and therapeutic dimension. What kind of knowledge is it?

Knowledge in medicine clearly possesses many dimensions other than the 'verified' and the 'unverified'. The quality of knowledge is characterized by, among other things, the form of responsibility that is typical for each of the modes of knowledge. Recognition of the particular form of responsibility is by no means a self-evident 'given', nor can the recognition process ever reach a final goal. It is one thing to know about the hereditary nature of a patient's tendency; another thing to know about the genetic impairment of one of his parents; a third thing to know about an injury to the patient during the foetal period; a fourth to know about a birth trauma; a fifth to know about the quality and phases of the patient's early nest; a sixth to know about the relations between the patient's mother and her mother-in-law; a seventh to know about the discriminations practiced in the patient's relevant community; an eighth to know about the causal thinking traditions; and so on. Knowledge that is directly therapeutic or methodical is also of many kinds: it is one thing to master the technical problems of a surgical operation; quite another to know the techniques of speech training; a third to provide care and restrictive guidance while simultaneously encountering the patient and his family empathetically and observing them (as ward nurses must do); and it is a fourth to surrender oneself to partnership with the patient in individual play therapy, in its various stages and dimensions. All this manifold methodical skill and knowledge is needed if other kinds of knowledge are to be given their 'natural' places. The approaches to the problems and qualities of the knowledge are also specifically dependent on which function of the team and which member are involved. Part of the knowing function belongs expressly to the team as a whole, and not to any of its members individually. Discussion and the associated *Besinnung* (penetration into oneself and the matter, and dwelling there) are also essential partial functions of the event of knowing. So is more general consideration of the information and insights gained, with a view to creating formulations with varying degrees of wider application, so that the experiences can be conveyed into the common fund.

Certain types of causes can only be encountered in a progressive process of therapy where gradual improvement involves both prolonged personal association with the patient and his family, and 'extended' responsibility. This particularly applies to encountering the patient's biographical causal network. In addition, however, numerous other 'factors' – cerebral damage, let us say, or the hereditary nature of an organic defect – acquire differentiated configurations only during prolonged, intensive, and personal therapeutic intercourse, in which one dimension of the therapeutic process is a continuous and progressive modification of the team's attitudes and approaches to the problem. Knowledge of causes varies with the quality, nature, and extent of the therapeutic responsibility acknowledged and 'lived through'. All causal inquiry takes us some way towards acknowledgement of responsibility, and yet away from it to some extent too. Clearly, a decisive point is whether the prevailing situation is one of struggle, or whether inertia has set in. The more our attitudes are controlled by (latently) despairing basic concepts, the greater our need to seek causes that will act as scapegoats: we try to make the causes into centres or objects where we can locate the dilemma, the distress, the anxiety, or our own existential debt,[1] and even our

---

[1] That is, one's own 'unlived life': the being that has not been fulfilled, or lived, in and through us, and thus weighs on us like an unpaid debt to life for what we have in turn received.

own share of the guilt. We are in flight. But from what? Experience in intensive individual therapy seems to suggest that there are certain common avoidances: we are in flight from a verdict of rejection by life, for example, which we unconsciously fear and expect. Another need to flee is from an emergence of life *in* and *for* us – which is seen as undeserved and thus experienced as a verdict about our ('empirical') self.

In other words, our concepts and doctrines concerning the causality of diseases are inevitably involved in the prevalent conflict over the freedom and servitude of man. Medical concepts and doctrines are an area of the battlefield; they are some of the results of the battle. Science, although often considered as such, is no neutral area. In science, however, it is as difficult as in international politics to make a neat distinction – a realistic one, that is – between the 'free' and 'totalitarian' worlds. The causal concepts held will not settle the distinction for us, though the attempt is sometimes made. All we can do is to assert that it is unmistakably important to acknowledge that in our pursuit of causes and in our causal doctrines we too are centrally entangled in man's basic dualities.

Similar considerations apply to the particular purposes for which causes are sought. In other words, how does the aim of our particular investigation, involving, as it will, a search for causes, shape our view of the disease configuration? One can visualize two distinct cases. Do those who are investigating and treating the patient visualize a given syndrome as a total 'actual disease configuration', whose correct diagnosis they must make? Or do they see the manifestation of the disease configuration as an unending process, in principle, appearing in association with a therapeutic encounter? In the latter case, every cause is a starting point for the next lap of the configuration's perpetually differentiating manifestation. Here, then, the responsible one or ones will not define in advance the dimensions that they agree to take into account in their search and consider relevant; they will not limit the dimensions into which the causes of the phenomena to be encountered are to be fitted.

The very directions in which causes are sought can also – and, one may suggest, should – be very diversified. 'Where is the cause?' The question clearly invites concrete details of space and time, but these can only be supplied in quite precisely limited connections. In the case of hoarseness, for instance, it is relevant to explicate several details: where and how the hoarseness was formed; when it was first observed to occur; and whether anything that can be considered the immediate cause of the hoarseness occurred then. But sometimes treatment of hoarseness proves a protracted and troublesome task. During speech therapy sessions, a natural, non-hoarse use of the voice is achieved over and over again. But for some reason – for what *cause?* – the patient makes no use of his skill outside the therapeutic sessions. Sometimes it then becomes obvious that the patient *needs* his speech impairment, because he can find no other excuse for, say, delaying his active grasp on life, on the way towards independence. The speech impairment perhaps prevents his participation in vocational training, or removes his possibilities of accepting a permanent opportunity of work. Hoarseness in a child, again, as with the hurried speech phenomenon in Chapter 2, can be the manifestation of a defect in the child's nest situation – one so massive that removal of the hoarseness, without first essentially correcting the nest situation, would inevitably lead the child to some more serious disorder than hoarseness. The configuration of speech impairment, the mere capacity or incapacity for articulated speech, does not as such reveal the nature of the total configuration; in itself it does not reveal the difficulty surrounding the patient's presence, of which the impairment forms a part. The total configuration will only gradually emerge in the therapeutic team's experience, in ever new dimensions, its aspects slowly and progressively becoming clearer. Moreover, every clarification will be followed by a relatively chaotic intermediate phase, before the picture becomes yet another degree more realistic.

In this process, the question of cause takes on many forms, many directions and several functions; and the question's very centre of gravity will have been transferred several times from one member of the team to another. Why are we keeping such a hopeless patient in the ward? Why is the patient so 'impossible' from this or that point of view? Why is it so difficult for me to tolerate his accentuated slowness of comprehension, his hearing difficulty with *my* speech in particular, his cajoling or his sadism? Why has the team, hitherto so patient, now turned almost unanimously against the child? Why do the ward nurse and the children's nurse nowadays always become argumentative when the talk turns to Pekka? The causal centre of gravity shifts from the patient to his family and other significant persons in his life, to the attitudes of society, to scientific concepts and prejudices, to individual members of the team, to inter-team relations, to the team as an entity, to the various aspects of the hospital community within the framework of which the team is working, and so on. The tone of the questions about cause ranges from panic, terror, anxiety, resignation, accusation, latent rejection, and ironic hardness to expectancy, curiosity, relevant observation, hope, euphoria and so on. Repeatedly the drift is towards the search for a scapegoat. In itself this will not be crucial, provided that, together, the team can continually reawaken to an insight into where things are going.

Answers to causal questions very rarely reveal themselves at the precise time when they are most needed. Only when it has been possible, without resignation, to remain with the question, when it has been possible to leave it open, will the answer emerge, perhaps through some unlooked-for personal channel. The question may be of the following sort, for instance. We are considering what aspects of the parents' relationship to our child-patient may have led to precisely *this* particular kind of speech shyness? Months of ward and play-therapy contacts have gone by, when we finally recognize that the patient's looks and postures have long been, as it were, trying to communicate to us: 'Yes – I ought to be all right now, oughtn't I, and speak the way you expect? But, of course, I *can't* do anything properly, can I? I'm no good, am I?' Probably we do not feel we have deserved this estimate of us. When, however, we are aware that we are irritated and impatient, we are simultaneously experiencing one aspect of the framework within which the relationship between this child and his parents clearly exists. It is not until we are forced to analyse this difficulty in ourselves that we can comprehend the question of cause in a more differentiated and relevant way.

IV   CAUSE AND EFFECT AS PROCESSES
OF VARIOUS DIMENSIONS; THE CAUSAL NETWORK

A therapeutic encounter 'with extended responsibility' is one where a *common* process of improvement is achieved in shared work between a team and the persons more particularly involved in the disease condition. Here a possibility gradually emerges of establishing contact with the constellation's network of causes and its history. Stage by stage, increasingly relevant causes are encountered. The causes, it becomes apparent, exert, and have exerted in certain past phases, an influence through certain particular channels, outlets, or hiatuses. The concept here stems from von Weizsäcker. Clearly, causal chains that are a tangle of human history and existential debt can have no unambiguous and clear-cut point of departure, or ultimate moment of onset. One can, however, follow, more or less clearly, how 'it' moves – or rather has moved – from one human being and state of existence to another. 'It' here is an element of sickness that has assumed a form but cannot be unambiguously defined. The movement occurs from generation to generation, from the community to the individual, from the individual to his organs.

During its transmission the element of sickness is transformed. There is, say, a distorted father-son relationship. In a certain stage of the boy's development the distortion is transformed into the boy's ardent and observable need to control all his reactions, even in their first incipient emotional stages. This boy's daughter, in turn, perhaps manifests 'it' as stuttering. In a still later phase 'it' perhaps moves into some individual's vocal cords or hearing organs. At the points of transition and transformation we can often identify the 'hiatuses' mentioned. Through a hiatus 'it' assumes a new state of existence, while the movement across the hiatus is often seen and felt as a disease process. The first 'hiatus' in our example was the development of the boy's self-control during childhood; the 'process' was the construction of the anxiety-defence system of a character neurosis. Subsequent *hiatuses* might be his marriage and the gene constellation created through the selection of a partner; here the *process* might be the congealment of the marital relationship into a pattern leading to the formation of a certain type of 'nest'. This 'nest' then provides the premises for the development of a special kind of self-control in the daughter's speech and this, in turn, for an individual with a certain potentiality, might provide a weighty incentive to stuttering.

An invented example like this only highlights a few of the innumerable circumstances and dimensions involved in the transmission and transformation, the hiatuses and processes, of an 'element of sickness'. The applications of the health/disease aspect to existence have been continually extended during the history of medicine. Yet only certain directions are recognized for causes of health and disease. And only certain types of transmission, transformation, hiatus, and process tend to be acknowledged as truly 'real'. In some way, too, it is still difficult for the immediately responsible ones in contemporary medicine to seriously consider anything but bodiliness, imagined as an object, as a substratum of disease. The tendency persists, though even a slightly more versatile examination and treatment of illness makes us encounter defects and disease phenomena as facts in the most diversified dimensions of shared existence. This is particularly conspicuous in cases of speech development disturbance. 'It' may be passing through, or lodged in, these dimensions as a more or less manifest process. The disease process is then both a distortion – within a certain dimension – and an attempt to avert distortion and disaster. As pointed out earlier, the further we are from accepting common responsibility for the dilemma, *human* responsibility, the more the dilemma becomes mechanical in its course: it follows its own laws and becomes more apparently an anonymous process. Cure, too, we must remember, proceeds through many hiatuses: cure is transmitted, transformed, and displays many facets of a process. These facets sometimes make it difficult – especially for an outsider – to realize that the direction *is* one of healing.

Here are a few examples of causal chains. Let us begin with Erik's grandmother. Her mothering 'caused' Erik's mother to hold a certain basic concept: that the grandmother's speech and the speech of adults in general represented *the* authentic picture and framework of reality. This young woman then became alienated from certain central features of her own being, and a crippling 'piousness' began to dominate her. This led, for instance, to helplessness about choosing a spouse – which, in turn, resulted in a very fragile nest and also great difficulty in preserving the foetus alive in the womb. The first pregnancy was molar. The delivery was then delayed and traumatic for the baby boy, who remained a stranger to his mother in many ways. This alienation pervaded the mother's relation to her son: it could be felt, for instance, in the way the mother discussed her son on her visits to the social worker. The transmission and transformation of the disease configuration could be schematized under the following sequence. First: the grandmother's domination – or distrust of the child's potentialities – and her belief in a monolithic world where might was alone right. Second: the mother's one-track speech control ('piousness'), her alienation in large parts of her being, incapacitating her for feelings of maternity, her importence to exercise choice concerning marital partner, the flimsy nest that resulted, the impaired 'hearing' of her child and her enfeeblement for mothering a child with cerebral injury. Third: the boy's birth trauma and his difficulties in controlling speech and voluntary movements.

In the case of Heikki, the corresponding sequence would be as follows. First: modern society's disorientated over-valuation of cash standards as the measure of 'standard of living'. Second: an *echo* of this common human impoverishment in the head of the family's standard-of-living psychosis, the wife's capitulation to it, and the consequent failure of her maternal capacities. Third: mere *echo*-speech in the child. A clearly important hiatus here was the mother-child relationship during the child's second and third years.

In the case of Raimo, again, only a shorter strip of the sequence was visible. First: a perverted concept of obedience in parents who were teachers, and an insistence on it. Second: the transformation of overcompliance into incapacity in the child's hearing organs. The hiatus here was the developmental stage of the obedience/independence dimension at the boy's age; the process was evidently a viral infection of the auditory nerve.

The reality of such sequences is hard to prove,[1] at least if the criteria are purely those of reductive control. If one participates in research and therapeutic work with extended responsibility, as for disturbances of speech development, one is most definitely confronted with the evident reality of these sequences. Yet it is difficult to reduce such an experiential world to a manageable conspectus, to make reductive controlling knowledge available. How could statistical proof of the most central circumstances be provided, for example? The mode of verification must, one would think, be correlated to the quality and nature of the experience. Clearly, in fact, the demand for statistical verifiability is not always appropriate. The fundamental insights, for instance, that form the necessary basis of the investigation are not amenable to statistical treatment. Typical insights of this sort might be the following: 'a human being behaves humanly even in his organs'; 'discrimination is one form of latent despair'; 'the psyche/soma alternatives only have a very limited relevance'; 'one of the most central problems in a therapy is the necessity of carrying it through, as far as possible, in a condition of abstinence' (S. Freud, 1919; see further below, p. 145; etc). But with disease constellations, too, it may take, say, three years of treatment before the team as a whole reaches a diagnostically identifiable configuration; during this period an average of three persons may devote themselves to the patient for an average of three hours each week. In such circumstances the demand for statistical verification appears problematic. There is probably an even more weighty consideration. Considering the multidimensionality of the individual histories, the possibilities of combination are so manifold that an

[1] The sequences outlined here are merely summary illustrative sketches; the details might be open to serious challenge, if offered as ultimate interpretations. Their function here is primarily to draw attention to the existence of such sequences and not to prove that the particular cases did have precisely these sequences beyond doubt.

attempt to collect a hundred statistically comparable cases would be unlikely to meet even partial success. The efforts made in this direction have, in fact, generally produced rather trivial results. There is an inverse ratio between extended responsibility in investigation and the feasibility of statistics. The more extended it is, the wider is the polarity between devotion and healing on the one hand and the systematic collection of data on the other. Information is, of course, obtained in abundance, but only a fragment of it is reducible to verified controlling knowledge. The more extended the responsibility, the greater is the information that escapes direct control as verified knowledge. In such a context, reductive control is revealed as but one among many ways of knowing and many types of responsibility: it becomes impossible to regard it as the criterion and model for estimating the validity of all knowledge.[1]

Now let us examine six cases of disturbed speech development. The causal network will be analysed on the basis of the case histories compiled by the other members of the team.

Petteri

On his first visit to the hospital Petteri was four and a half years old. On his second visit, he was one year older. At the first encounter in the clinic the child was considered hard-of-hearing. The parents' central reason for complaint was his speechlessness. Both the boy's upper lids were found to be ptotic; no hearing deficiency, nor anything else specific, was establishable at this time. On his second visit Petteri no longer had even the rhinitis that had been present previously. The mother had given birth to Petteri, who was her only child, at the age of thirty-eight. The child was delivered by caesarean section, whereupon a depression was observed in his forehead; this subsequently disappeared. Petteri was a lazy breast-feeder and vomited quite a lot. In the first two months of his life he was very restless. He was not toilet-

[1] Clearly, the critical screening of all insights and knowledge that do not come fully, or even at all, into the category of reductive controlling knowledge is a duty and a problem. Consideration of this must, however, be postponed for a further study.

trained until the age of three. In other respects – apart from the speech development – the child's early development showed no unusual features, in the opinion of the parents. At the age of four the boy had learned to say: 'Give! Mine! Mummy! Skirt!' At the time of the child's birth and subsequently, the family shared a joint household with the father's family. The mother had been very distressed about her child. In the ward Petteri proved incoherent and lacked concentration; he was fanatically orderly and enjoyed teasing other children. The psychological tests revealed underdevelopment in static control and co-ordinatory control of the body. On the other hand Petteri's bearing in the ward was like that of the proprietor of a large farming estate. His mother also said that the boy was very eager to be with adults when they were working and learn how to do the jobs; he also understood orders and prohibitions. (The boy's object of identification was perhaps his grandfather, the master of the joint household, for the essence of 'the boss' could be recognized in Petteri.)

A total picture, a basic diagnosis, began to form from the data: his malleable mother, unable to assume her share of the living human space; his father, who did not recognize that a task confronted him – to form his own family into a specific unit distinct from the general 'family jelly' – and did not even recognize the problem. Since the child's nest was not distinguished from the surrounding world, from the grandfather's family, which was the father's own nest-space, it was difficult for Petteri to develop into a speaking centre, for his own family, and particularly his mother, had 'nothing to say' there. (In its basic pattern this resembles Eero's constellation, described in the first chapter.) As to his intellectual talents, no definite information was obtained; but the tests suggested that the boy's prerequisites should have been adequate for even a considerable ability to speak. Was Petteri's underdeveloped physical control an element of a general immaturity, including speaking impairment? Or was it rather the partial cause of the latter? The spouses' late marriage and their late child-bearing, on the other hand, certainly reflected the immaturity that was revealed in their inability to distinguish themselves from their environment in the father's family house. The possible birth trauma, again, was obviously associated with the primipara's relatively advanced age; and the same maternal tardiness was probably operative in the mother's defective ability to create a nest for her baby. Phenomenologically, the case could be characterized as follows: the span between the point 'skirt' (one of Petteri's first words) and the point 'boss' (the boy's essence in the ward) was too great: and there were no materials for constructing a bridge over the span. (In this respect, Petteri calls to mind the hero of Günther Grass's novel *The Tin Drum*.)

Petteri's treatment would have necessitated help for his parents. Motivation would have been necessary for their prolonged cooperation with the psychologist and the social worker, so that improvement in the condition of their nest could take place. There were, however, too many simultaneous obstacles blocking such attempts: they couldn't start on the path. To begin with, our medical tradition is not accustomed to seeing the tasks in this light. Thus, the members of the team who recognized this kind of problem could not obtain sufficient support for such intervention, nor the practical facilities. In addition, Petteri's father gave the impression of being completely unaware, entirely unawakened, concerning the basic factors of the situation, and the mother was almost entirely so. Thus, even to initiate co-operation would have been a problem – though perhaps a realizable project if the parents had encountered basic unanimity of attitude in all their contacts at the clinic; or if an authoritative source had not given them strong support for locating the entire dilemma in a defectiveness of their son. The latter tendency exists, in fact, in all of us; it is more prevalent in some people than in others, but nevertheless it is present in everyone on occasion. But the situation is particularly unfavourable if a strong mesh of the causal network is the clinic's own prevailing authoritative and accepted view of disease – if the disease is virtually unambiguously located by the clinic in objective causes and processes.

According to Viktor von Weizsäcker, the founder of 'anthropological medicine', bodily illness occurs as a substitute for thinking not brought to completion and for unacted basic human decisions.[1] In the case of Petteri, the substitute illness had become the lot of the child, as is very often the case. The very conception of a child is of a being that lives in and through his parents; and the smaller or more immature the child is, the more is this true. As regards his less developed features, the child is entirely dependent on his parents.

Eino

And then there is Eino: a four-year-old boy. His hearing was found to be mildly defective; his acoustic discrimination was observed to be disturbed as well, and (in association with the latter) so was his concentration, but not his motor functions. As to his intelligence, Eino gave the impression of being somewhat below average. The boy did not speak at all, but he did make himself understood to some extent by means of sign language, and he skilfully imitated animals' cries.

The child's birth was twelve days overdue, but nevertheless he only weighed 2·5 kg. His early development (apart from that of speech) was described as normal by the mother. At about the age of one-and-a-half to two years Eino suffered from otitis media, which healed well. Had this possibly been accompanied by encephalitis? The anamnestic data remained deficient in this respect. The mother was eighteen years old when she married, and by now she had four children, the eldest of whom was five. Eino was the second in order, and the remaining children were girls. Two of them, met at the clinic, seemed normally developed. The mother said the boy was jealous of his sisters, whom he angrily tried to control 'like children generally do'. This, as will be remembered, also occurred in the case of Petteri. If a child cried, Eino might be moved to come for help, although otherwise he teased other children, evidently enjoying their reactions.

Obviously, in some part of himself, the boy instinctively perceived that continued residence in the ward would be vitally important for him, for he fell ill with fever after he heard that his mother was coming to take him away. The mother, who lived

[1] Cf. Hübschmann (1963).

in a remote district, was in fact, acting against the advice of the personnel in doing so. Perhaps she had anticipated that she could bear no more light to be thrown on her family situation.

Actually, in this case, a contributory cause of the speechlessness (in fact its structural element) was some degree of acoustic agnosia. What *that* was – what stage of what process of non-integration – was not evident from the case history. This agnosia did not occur for animal sounds. Here the sparse speech development might be, in part, a manifestation of oligophrenia as well. It would have been important, from the point of view of the boy's future, to clarify this point. The boy's basic discontent, which took the form of jealousy, for instance, and a sadistic relation to other children, indicated that he felt some unrealized potentialities in himself. The mother was also clearly dissatisfied, but not in an active or hopeful way. She was inclined to tears, and her only immediate protest against her own situation was encountered as an exceptionally powerful odour of perspiration. Early marriage, with rapidly recurring pregnancies, is often a manifestation of some form of escape. At the same time it effectively absorbs the woman in actual care, thus assisting her to avoid surveying the situation as a whole. As to the boy's father and the interrelationship between the spouses, not much information was gained. This family, then, displayed its distress in one way, but at the same time also concealed it. At any rate it was not yet ready to penetrate into its own situation together with the team. How far would the team have been prepared to go in this direction, as an entity? Its own situation, immersed in our scientific medical and therapeutic tradition, did not encourage very free or intensive engagement, except in a few cases. However that may be, Eino's examination and treatment remained badly incomplete; thus the picture of his disease constellation also remained fragmentary.

Aarne

The diagnosis of nine-year-old Aarne was sigmatismus interdentalis, rhotacismus, hypertrophia tonsillae pharyngae (abrasio). Was there a cerebral lesion? In the psychological tests the boy's IQ was found to be 113; he was discovered to have difficulties with visual discrimination, and his motor development was established as one-and-a-half years below the norm for his age level. Since the EEG was also definitely abnormal and asymmetric, it was concluded that there was a mild cerebral injury. Aarne was able to concentrate well, but he proved stereotypical, shy, and withdrawing. In school and in speech therapy, however (or 'therefore'?), he was a good student.

His mother had given birth to him prematurely, but his birth weight was normal. The essential information, however, was that the mother's menstrual periods continued, recurring regularly, throughout the pregnancy. The team noted that the mother observably adhered to her son with severe feelings of guilt. Aarne was permitted to dominate his mother at will, and the boy had learned this lesson so well that he even succeeded in tyrannizing over the nurses in the ward. Clearly the continuance of her menstrual periods throughout pregnancy indicated that the boy's mother had, with some element in her, quite radically denied the reality of her pregnancy. A corresponding manifestation of attitude at the psychic level is sometimes encountered: a woman comes to the doctor and complains of an abdominal tumour, assuring him that she has never had anything to do with men, while she is really already in the late stages of pregnancy, and the foetus may even have been moving in her womb for several months.

In this case, too, then, the case history yielded suggestions in a certain direction – which, for one reason or another, were not followed up and investigated. Elucidation of the family dynamics, and thus of Aarne's nest situation, consequently remained incomplete, although many other facts were rather fundamentally registered. Such facts, however, remain disconnected if there is no firm total therapeutic grasp.

Toivo

The diagnosis of seven-year-old Toivo was dysphasia, dysgrammatismus, dysarthria, (dysphonia), deficientia intelligentiae. The EEG report referred, with interrogation marks, to disturbances of myelinization; the report concluded with the diagnosis:

dysfunctio atypica (macrorhythmia) et dysrhythmia epileptica atypica regionis occipitalis l.a. This boy had attended the ordinary elementary school up to the third grade, but this can only be explained through the unsatisfactoriness of the facilities for special education in many parts of Finland. (This is partly due to the large geographical distances involved.)

Toivo was a big boy who proved very obedient in the ward; psychological examination failed to show any 'emotional difficulties'. This raised a question. Where did his balance come from? Was it defective intelligence that made the boy content with his situation? Was it the attitude of his parents? Or what? The father seemed to have been unaware of his son's developmental defect, but the mother seemed to have had some notion of it. Neither of them had considered their son mentally retarded. Were the parents themselves scarcely differentiated, intellectually? Were their child's resources, perhaps, essentially better manifested at home than in the ward? Or did the parents for some reason reject the reality of their child's developmental defect from their minds?

Here, too, the mother was pregnant while the couple were living with the man's parents. During much of the pregnancy there had been no speech between the mother-in-law and the daughter-in-law. This fact was in the case history, but there had been no progression beyond this, no clarification as regards the kind of constellation involved, of which this fact would form a part. The picture of the phenomenon that seemed to emerge from the case history raised the following question. Was the lack of integration in the poisonous marriage situation left to be the burden of the unborn child? Apparently, there was no space for expressing the distress that existed on the psychic level: in fact, precisely this distress was taboo for some reason. Perhaps ruptures of reciprocal comprehension at the technical level – not only hearing defects but also impediments in the speech-instrument – often serve a vital protective function: they shield children from tasks that are completely beyond the powers of a growing infant to perform alone – tasks supposed to be performed vicariously for adults.

In this case too it is observable how scanty is the functional and therapeutic potential of exact objective registrations, if they are not allowed articulation within a broader and more comprehensive grasp, where they can assume their own place.

Vesa

Vesa, an orphanage child aged seven and a half, spoke unclearly and could not pronounce r or s. The boy, the second of his mother's three illegitimate children, was born prematurely, and weighed 1·7 kg. His tonsils were found to be hypertrophied, and he was said to have had tonsillitis quite often. (According to von Weizsäcker, tonsillitis is generally connected with separation and detachment in situations that are beyond the individual's powers of acknowledgement and appropriation – and still less assimilation.) The boy's intelligence was of low average level, his verbal and motor development below average. Vesa was incoherent, had a short attention span, and was, according to the psychologist's statement, immature. In his case, however, the EEG report said nothing about disturbance of myelinization, only mentioning bradyrhythmia diffusa. According to data obtained from the orphanage, the boy's early development had been normal apart from speech. He started to speak at the age of three. He clearly became more lively in the ward – in an environment providing more incentives. He then proved capable of both initiative and sensible opposition.

The central issue here too was 'early separation' – separation at an early age from the nest provided by the mother. A special feature of Vesa's situation was the 'rejecter's' entire disappearance from the child's range of vision. This was not the case with, for example, Pentti, Heikki, and Lauri. Vesa's mother gave her son to the orphanage and then never asked about him afterwards. 'Early separation' actually only arises when there is no effective substitute for the mother. Clearly the orphanage had, in this case, provided a substitute nest in some degree, since the child's speech had at least partly developed. Vesa's case revealed a pervasive defectiveness of incentives for development.

Early separation is well documented: it has been shown how greatly all the mental and physical partial phenomena of a child's development depend on fundamental factors of the nest constellation. Among others, Spitz (1945) and Bowlby (1951) have performed thoroughgoing investigations in a framework of extensive series. Nevertheless early separation is only one extreme and specific form of deprivation. The same basic structure is characteristic of all human growth and development, as the observations made about early separation conclusively prove. And yet, when dealing with other phenomena of deprivation, we go on abstracting ourselves from our insights into human prerequisites: we ignore the humanity of the sick person, ignoring radical human dependencies, which are facts, ignoring the basic existential prerequisites of man's being.

Keijo

In the case of six-year-old Keijo, the intricate structure of the intertwined causes seems to emerge with particular clarity. The operative factors appear in all their multimodality. The boy's speech was to some extent agrammatical, and the r and the s were defective. Keijo's intelligence was of a good average level, but his motor functions were clumsy, and both his auditory and his visual discrimination were distinctly defective. The EEG revealed dysrhythmia diffusa (organica?) et tachyrhythmia (e medicam.?); there was dysrhythmia epileptica paroxysmalis subcorticalis.

Slow development of speech had occurred in the family; in addition, all three of Keijo's sisters only learned to speak after the age of two. One of the sisters was defective in speech in a way similar to Keijo. After the accidental death of one of Keijo's sisters in a road accident, one year before Keijo's birth, his mother had an ovarian tumour. One of the mother's sisters had had breast cancer; the mother's father had had laryngeal carcinoma; and even her grandfather had had some kind of carcinoma. Keijo's father – according to the data provided by the mother – was pathologically jealous. (For comparison, the parents of a patient in our phoniatric ward both gave this estimate of each other.)

Keijo was born past term; his head was severely elongated, and he had to be kept in an oxygen incubator. The data about his early development are as follows. The boy was walking at the age of thirteen months and was toilet-trained after fifteen months. After he was two, he was able to use some words, but these were later forgotten. Stomach-ache and vomiting were frequent. When he was quite young, Keijo was an 'exceptionally nice boy' – who had temper-tantrums at times, 'however', whereupon he turned bluish and was driven to blind violence. In the ward the boy teased other children and refused to eat.

Turning now to the complex of causes, we find the following. There was a family tendency towards delayed speech development; the postmaturity of Keijo's birth; a birth trauma and asphyxia; EEG symptoms; and indications of cerebral defect, or damage, or both, taking the form of defective general perception and control. A factor that influenced both his general development and his speech was that he could find no place in himself for anger – or any opposition or frustration reactions in general – except through attacks of rage that made him breathless. His refusal to eat in the ward, taking the boy's age into account, reflected a fundamental insecurity, so great that it understandably prevented him from experiencing even the safe aspects of his ward environment: the dominant fact in the situation for him was that arrival at the ward was a *change*, and change represented the immediate threat of catastrophe for this child. In his case, then, the trend towards orderliness (the early toilet-training) represented adaptation to an environmental rhythm that others imposed, exacted, and expected. The adaptation had not become integrated into the entity. Keijo had not grown to appreciate and foster his own interests through increasingly differential measures: he had felt forced to allow infringements of his rights, until frustration prompted release in fits of rage.

Keijo's difficulties in speech appeared to be, at least in part, components of his dysrhythmia in breathing, in excretion, and in elementary and necessary self-expression. How did all this fit into the boy's family constellation? How had this stage been reached in the hereditary constellations, in the hereditary events, in the maternity crises of Keijo's mother, in the stages of her pregnancy, in the event of delivery, and in the child's early development? What place and share, here, were occupied by the accidental death of Keijo's sister, by the mother's ovarian tumour, and, finally, by the father's jealousy? All these are not, of course, necessarily associated with Keijo's speech problems. In the phoniatric ward the configuration of Keijo's constellation remained very fragmentary for the team. A wider and deeper disentanglement of such a constellation and such a causal network can only, in general, be achieved during intensive and prolonged therapy for both the child and his family. The therapy must be able (and must be allowed) to advance on all the fronts where resistance to improvement is essentially encountered.

How do these six cases illuminate the chain of causality in disturbances of speech development? At least they disclose that various kinds of obstacles and resistances obstruct the disentanglement of causes, and that many prerequisites must be fulfilled before relevant progress can take place. The parents' unawareness, their ambivalence or attitude of rejection towards the difficult child – these are often condensed into an impenetrable resistance; particularly so if there is a great distance between the place of residence and the phoniatric ward and this can be used to excuse the reduction of work with the difficulties to a minimum. There are other contributory factors: these often include the attitudes of the medical and social officials in the family's place of residence, and also the attitudes of the neighbourhood. Consciousness of illness, the recognition and admission that there is distress and need of treatment, always has a communal aspect, extending beyond the limits of the family. On the other hand, these six cases also reveal that the arrest of disentanglement in certain phases was connected with the investigational and therapeutic team's own unawareness and inexperience; apparently the team sometimes faltered, and faith broke down, when the network of causes appeared excessively complicated. This again had something to do with the pioneering nature of the struggle and the scarcity of support from the immediate environment. Thus, it is broadly true to say that, up to now, the present team has been unable to reach a clear and unanimous conviction about the true significance of all the causal dimensions touched upon above.

V MAN AS THE RECEIVER OF MAN
UNREALIZED POTENTIALITIES: GUILT, SICKNESS, AND DEFECT AS SECURITIES FOR THE DEBT OF UNLIVED LIFE

The history of every individual, like the history of every community, is a history of receiving and being received. The whole history specifically has the configuration of receiving, and each constituent situation in the history also has the specific configuration of receiving. A *history* is a relation to man, to a human community – whether understood as a 'group' or an 'organism' – and to human potentialities; and it is in receiving and being received that we live out the human – our relationship to the image of man – the image of man that each person experiences others and himself to be. The reception experienced by every child – his 'receiving world' – may be outlined from various angles, but one important angle is that the reception has a long historical dimension: any reception is the result of a long process, created individually and collectively. A receiving-process has an aim: living that is specifically human. This is true of every phase in the being of man, of every formative stage: heredity, conception, pregnancy, delivery, early and later infancy, school age and prepuberty, puberty, adolescence, adulthood, middle age, senescence, and so on – these are 'human'. All these phases are conducted in the 'atmosphere' of our preconceptions, though some are more responsibly acknowledged than others. The events are shot through with our basic views and beliefs – and also with *our* passivity. They are permeated with both our ideologies and *our* despair, *our* freedom and *our* dependence, *our* tradition and *our* chaotic 'drives'.

All causes, whether comparatively objectified and verified or beyond computation, are realized – thus, occur – in the specific unity that is *human* existence: in the manifold, but always in some way defined and characteristic, dimensions of this whole complex. Thus the causes of human diseases and defects cannot ever be entirely beyond human responsibility and guilt. They are inseparable from man's obligation to his life for his specific being, his indebtedness. The spatially and temporally specified causal events that we have verified are always *selections*. They have been isolated from the wider historical configurations of certain dimensions of human existence. These wider configurations must, however, be brought into view if we wish to set a healing process in motion – a new integration, and not the mere elimination of a narrowly defined defect, curtailed in both space and time.

Traditionally, medicine has tended to favour two stands concerning cause: either the cause is an unchanged and unchangeable irreversibility; or it is an eradicable defect, an evil that has been unearthed from concealment and must be removed from the scene. The causes whereby diseases and defects originate and are maintained are not readily seen as containing any hidden productive possibilities. And yet the experience in extended, long-term treatment makes it increasingly clear that a substantial improvement always means more than the mere disappearance of some defect or detriment: it means the discovery of sources and potentialities that were previously concealed. The essence of cure is the emergence of some aspect of individual and communal life, and its unfolding process of realization. The causes of the diseases and defects of an existing human being always reveal themselves as involved with human guilt. Neglected possibilities, unlived individual and collective life, unintegrated potentialities – a man feels guilty because of these. He feels them as an 'unpaid debt' – a failure to respond to life with life, to pay his potentialities into the fund of life that he has drawn on. This existential guilt, this sense of an unpaid debt, is signalized through 'causes' of disease and disturbance, which are the manifestations of unlived life, unpaid debts, guilt. But, as such, they have a positive aspect. Amidst all the factual devastation, unused resources are at stake and are suggested by the situation. There is an implication of talents, possibilities, reserves, potentialities, and, as it were, treasures that have partly remained unrealized and even been partly destroyed. Now they are indicated, there is the possibility of their being realized. The productive possibilities of defects and diseases are, however, realized in surprising ways and unexpected dimensions. Often, perhaps mostly, the realization occurs unrecognized.

Let us consider an example. Suppose that the absoluteness of Pentti's isolation is broken; progressive reciprocal comprehension begins to occur, even though Pentti does not learn articulated speech to a significant degree. In such circumstances, it may be that something is becoming essentially integrated in the *team*: even more, a new insight is being achieved which will lead to new and productive hypotheses concerning children's speech impairments. If so, these gains could be said to constitute part of the process of Pentti's disease and cure. But we are likely to overlook the part Pentti's disease has played in releasing these potentialities in others. Traditionally, we are accustomed to viewing the substrata of disease, defects, and cure in a different manner.

VI THE BASIC ANTHROPOLOGICAL CHANNEL OF CAUSATION IN DEFECTS AND DISEASES

To conclude this chapter, there follows a brief summary of the conception preliminarily mentioned at the end of Chapter 2: the fundamental pattern or basic aetiological model of causation, as I see it. This is the process of *vicarious* illness: the organ suffers instead of the organism; the individual suffers instead of the community. 'Instead', in this connection, implies that the individual's own responsibility and the community's collective responsibility have remained partially unrealized. Proper understanding of the following summary would actually require acquaintance with certain sections of my book *Die Schizophrenie – des Einzelnen und der Allgemeinheit* (Schizophrenia – in the Individual and the Community). The account is nevertheless appended here for the sake of systematic completeness.

The causality of illness is seen as proceeding along a basic channel characteristic of man's existence. One aspect of the channel is illustrated by the following model.

Let us begin with what may be described as 'primary legalism'. This includes a delusion of primary autonomy, which is the misconception that one is the ultimate judge of good and evil – that one has the ultimate criteria for judging what is encountered in life, in oneself, in one's fellow-men and in the world. This involves 'bad conscience' – for one judges oneself – despair and suspicion. These, in turn, stop one receiving what is encountered; they also bring along an absolutist primary aspiration towards mastery, or at least control, of the life one suspects and despairs of. This is 'primary legalism'.

This fundamental human misconception – the delusion of being the knower of good and evil – has been the matrix in which various problems have matured: tangles of delusion, stemming from both historical traditions and contemporary existence; unrealized debts to life; 'blinding' vendetta-sequences; failure of integration; tangled networks of wrong; and the bitterness of those who are tangled up in them.

In a situation such as this, one causal channel becomes illness: in other words, a substitute event. In a particular crisis the tangle, though a communal one, is not recognized or acknowledged as a common responsibility – by emerging, for example, into common consciousness; 'instead' illness takes its place. Shared consciousness is only possible if the power of despair can be broken to an extent: so far, at least, as to prevent doctrines of despair inhibiting the encounter with the essential challenges and resisting the formation of the relevant approaches.

Vicarious illness – the individual suffering instead of the community, the organ suffering instead of the organism – is nevertheless a form of address: it is a substitute for shared conscious responsibility, but it nevertheless reaches out towards it. The language employed is, for instance, the allegorical statement of a psychosis; or a speech even more remote from articulated speech, a code of the organs.

In every phase of a causal process there are two basic directions and basic possibilities: either the appeal will be left out of account, or it will sooner or later be heard. Either the appeal will progressively go underground – farther from reciprocal comprehensibility – or the appeal will be received into joint responsibility, approaching human articulation, which may increase progressively in a search for shared responsibility and the realization of unlived life. Let us put the two side by side.

The process has a growing adherence to its own laws, and thus appears to be mechanically determined. The process is moulded in accordance with a predictable disease-picture. Destruction of organs takes place, and there is havoc in the I–me and I–thou relationships. The patient appears to be the helpless victim of an anonymous fate. Despair is reinforced in the patient, the medical staff, and the patient's family. Evidence appears to have been provided for a mechanically determined course of events. The patient, the family, the medical staff, and thus the community are impoverished because potentialities in all of them are denied emergence.

Transference takes place. The problem received in substitute-form is transferred from the organ to the sphere of common responsibility: from the organ to the organism and from the individual to joint communal responsibility.[1] Transformation of a symptom takes place in the direction of the realization of unlived life as integrated forms: denied potentialities are integrated into the organism, the community, the world and life. This is the reverse of mechanical determination, adhering to it own laws. The course is towards man's freedom, which is realized when the life in him establishes communal and personal reference. Thus the appeal that is the disease can here lead to encounters in which health emerges from disease and the individual and the community are enriched: enrichment is 'caused'.

[1] Here again, appropriation of individual personal responsibility can occur.

CHAPTER 4

Analysis of some Key Concepts

I PSYCHE/SOMA THINKING:
THE UNDIFFERENTIATED BASIC BIPOLAR PATTERN

As established above, our search for causation often becomes, quite primarily, restricted within concepts of reductive control. However, many things that will not fit into this framework nevertheless force themselves on us as significant causes, and one traditional solution to this problem has been to extend the area of reference a little by taking so-called 'psychic factors' into account. An attempt is made to observe these concurrently with organic factors, or as continuations of organic factors, though this is done hesitantly and in some ways in isolation from the accepted scientific system. The connecting links between psychic and organic factors are taken to be the vegetative nervous system, the endocrine system, and certain cerebral structures. In certain limited connections this procedure is, in fact, clearly relevant; but it scarcely fulfils the requirements of a scientific system. Reenpää's analysis, quoted above, showed that the concepts we use in exact research are constructed out of the 'material' of our elementary sensory experiences. This reveals one of the fundamentally problematic aspects of the traditional procedure. For the exact concepts whereby we characterize the organic and the somatic are in fact themselves 'psychic', if we remain within the two alternatives.

The mode of thought that operates with the two alternatives, somatic and psychic factors in combined pairs, is obviously based on materialist metaphysics (or alternatively on the spiritualist counterpart), with roots going far back into our history. Yet there is some ambiguity involved here. Even since the time of Einstein

96

and Planck materiality has been experienced in science in terms of various notions of energy (or energy in terms of matter). On the other hand we are increasingly able to extend exact methods for the description of the most spiritual activities. Nevertheless we still cling to our illusion that materiality is in some way given, as if it were the most real basis of existence. Here, in fact, we are not very far from the (magic) conception that the existent most immediately perceptible to the senses[1] is the most real; and that this, as something immediately given, contains the basic causes of the structure of reality.

This is connected with a tradition that burdens medicine: the concept that the essence of the soma and the somatic is, in fact, material. Materiality, again, is imagined as self-evidently given in one's perception. Materiality is evidenced as, say, solidity or self-contained compactness. And yet the essence of the soma, of bodiliness, includes, among other things at least, a living integratedness into a human organism, concentrated in time. When matter is being integrated into an organism, it is as remote as possible from its self-contained, compact, solid essence: through the most delicate strands and manifold adjustments, it is being integrated into the entity of an organism as its structures and functions, and finally into the existence of a human individual. It is as a being that has transcended itself historically, and is currently transcending itself, into human existence that matter reveals itself – *geht auf* – yields its essence. Only when man is dying – dying as a total human entity and dying as his human organs – does matter approach self-contained compact being and enter into a more mechanical course, with its own laws and the predictability characteristic of various material processes. And yet, even then, when the body is decomposing, matter is again becoming integrated into new areas of life and growth, in becoming nutritional and structural parts of living organisms.

[1] Living our lives almost exclusively supported by direct touch or – as is largely the case in modern society – technical controllability, it is quite natural that the most real aspect of existing is, for us, that which can be touched or controlled. When other kinds of existents in our reality also attempt to penetrate into the sphere of our consciousness, their eventual uncontrollability intimidates us into despairing endeavours to maintain our metaphysics, our view of life, intact.

The being of organs and organisms, as specialized structures serving special purposes, is an expression of bodiliness as integration. Every organ, in fact, is, lives, and becomes realized in many different basic ways and in the most manifold structural and functional dimensions. The organs are at once autonomous, in the service of other organs and dependent on other organs. An organ is built up subject to the overall developmental process of the total entity. An organ limits itself and creates boundaries against the surrounding tissues and organs. It has close and distant contacts. There are both microscopic and macroscopic 'influences'. The organ participates in the whole organism's defence systems and also has methods of defence more specifically for itself. It directs and is itself subject to direction. And so on.

Also, the organ participates in any of the organism's existence that concerns its own sphere. It does so in accordance with its own nature and the quality of its tasks. The digestive system, for instance, participates in breaking down, digesting and utilizing everything it takes in, in neutralizing dangerous elements and excreting poisonous and waste products. The same organ system is also always 'tuned-in', as it were, whenever the individual's total situation includes taking in, breaking down, etc., even if literal food is not actually in question.[1] To the degree that the total organism is unable to respond to the challenges personally and with full responsibility in its own dimension, the pressure of the challenges is passed on. The pressure becomes the burden of the organ system in one way or another. The vital integration that constitutes healthy order is then threatened, and there is an imminent possibility that the dilemma will materialize as an organic process. The process thus becomes more self-containedly 'material' – it operates more in terms of the laws inherent in 'materiality' – the more remote the possibility is of the total organism responding to the challenge in *human* terms: in terms of personal responsibility – 'spiritually', in other words. Contrariwise, the realization of the spirituality of man always constitutes some integration into the human community and into the larger, shared world.[2] The destructive direction of the process can

---

[1] See, for example, Boss (1954).   [2] See above, p. 57.

thus be characterized under the following scheme. There is a passage of responsibility, onwards and downwards. What begins as a communal responsibility is passed on to an individual to become his personal responsibility. Thence it becomes an anonymous individual responsibility and finally the responsibility of an organ. This means that the disease is increasingly becoming a material process, obeying more and more its own laws, as common human responsibility and reality are progressively denied.

In this light, the classification into psychic, somatic or organic has a merely limited value as a medical orientation: it is only of use for *ad hoc* decisions. Why is this boy crying so bitterly? Is it because he has been hit on the head while playing cricket? Or is the main point that he has been humiliated and is suffering about it? Does the patient now require a thorough examination – from a neurological point of view, for example? Or is he in need of a few sympathetic words? Perhaps he needs psychiatric treatment – since his response to the experience of humiliation is so radical? For a situation of this kind, application of the psyche/soma alternatives is adequate enough, but the significance and justification of the procedure does not seem to go deeper. In more differentiated contexts, the bipolar concept 'psyche/soma' rarely seems to point to anything real – except our thought fossils. All man's existence is, after all, in some way physical and organic. We need more, then, than a mere psyche/soma classification. We need to recognize innumerable nuances of the humanly organic, its modes of disintegration, and its possibilities of reconstruction.

Historically, research, the acquisition of knowledge, and systematic control of nature and human nature, were long obstructed by complaisance to the magical and static canon of philosophico-theological 'certain' knowledge, to be taken on trust in terms of 'faith'. Thus, during the centuries of science a firm reaction took place: the person emboldened to experimental research was unwilling to accept as truly relevant knowledge anything that did not lead to generally valid, systematic control of all the existents encountered. In other words, he would only accept reductive controlling knowledge. Yet, as pointed out above, consideration of the so-called 'psychic' factors did disturb the system's supposition of exactitude and general validity. Freud was aware of this. He was the first to elucidate the significance of 'psychic factors' in illness, systematically and in a consistently relevant way. Yet he continued to expect that, within the framework of the therapeutic method he called psychoanalysis, future science would provide more than the provisionally useful 'psychic factors'. There would, he thought, be a return to 'firm ground' in the form of physico-chemical facts.

As demonstrated previously, Reenpää's conceptual analysis and von Weizsäcker's anthropological medicine (to say nothing of the developments in the exact sciences themselves during recent decades) reveal the inapplicability of such an expectation. There is, in fact, no sure basic reality, either physical or otherwise. Research in the exact sciences is leading us in quite the contrary direction. It is working towards a conceptual differentiation that continually moves away from palpability, compact self-containedness, solidity, and all the traditional patterns of imagery specifically applied to 'matter'. Nor do psychic factors, as contrary and complementary concepts to those of somatic-materiality, hold up under criticism. How could they be applied, for example, to human speech where a voice – operating via a space satellite, say – addresses a fellow creature on the other side of the globe? Is the speech in this case psychic or organic? The artificiality of the entire mode of thought is demonstrated by a question such as this. Nor is the situation improved if, while restricting oneself within these narrow concepts, one argues that the psyche and the soma are the same thing, two aspects of the same thing, and so on. The dimensions of man's being are too numerous, his modes of existence and integration are too varied, and they are structured in terms of too many diversified categoric relationships, for any such bipolar conceptualism to suffice for differentiated purposes.

And yet research is still burdened and enmeshed by a conceptual constellation like this. For example, Arnold[1] (1960) writes: 'it [tachyphemia] represents an organically determined limitation in

[1] The author mentioned is an expert in phoniatrics with a wide international reputation. The contents of the footnote on p. 66 are fully applicable here too.

cerebral language function. Emotional and other purely psychological causes can safely be excluded.' Let us recall here that Freud, who was one of the great initiators of the crisis in the medical image of man, himself rejected, in 1933, von Weizsäcker's proposal that an infectious organic process (tonsillitis) could have underlying 'non-somatic' causes. At that time the conception of somatism was still so firmly bound to the accepted traditional imagery concerning materiality that even Freud was unable at this point to detach himself from the accustomed ways of thinking. Conceptually, the body and its materiality remained a somatic area even for von Weizsäcker (who was inspired by Freud). But in spite of this, on the basis of his clinical experience, he established that the body was part of a wider order of existence. For von Weizsäcker, the soma reflects human and spiritual modes of existence, the living and the non-living in humanity, in all their hierarchical multifariousness: during disease, the soma and its organs begin to speak instead of the individual or the community; they deputize for the psyche and the *Geist*. Surely the psyche/soma mode of thinking that has characterized the whole bygone age is now thoroughly out of date. Obviously we must get rid of it completely so that we can be liberated for a more realistic and fertile study and understanding of man in his manifold existential modes. This recognition of complexity and reality is particularly urgent for medical science. The reduction of reality to this simplified bipolarity can no longer possess the dignity of science.

Let us consider, for example, existential dimensions such as these: being a child, and being a parent; being a man, and being a woman; being nourished, and nourishing somebody else; comprehensibility to oneself, and the comprehensibility of fellowmen to each other; the unfolding of the world and life to a man; the zoomorphic aspects of man in the light of various categories and species of animals, certain factors of development, and so on; being accepted and making one's own contribution to and impression on the common world; participation in intimate spheres, and public intercourse; manifesting rhythm, music, the fine arts, co-operation and competition, rest and restlessness, work, hurry and destruction, growth and stagnation, play and athletic sports, learning and forgetting. It does not matter which of these are selected as 'psychic' or 'somatic', even for the sake of example: a statement in these terms would either be invalid or say virtually nothing. And yet the encounter with 'being ill' in terms of examination and treatment, even in the description of symptoms, must also necessarily move in some of these dimensions. *We are healthy and sick* in all of these dimensions. The conceptual, intellectual and linguistic habits that have deep roots in our history inhibit us from moving freely and without prejudice in the area of disease. In this way innumerable dimensions, not only of disease but of research and treatment, are excluded from observation and concern.

But where, it may be asked, shall we arrive if the psyche/soma pattern is abandoned and medicine agrees to move in the multiple dimensions of human existence? Will it be possible to establish any order in such an unlimited multiplicity? There seem to be good reasons for exposing ourselves to this difficulty. The other alternative, in fact, would be the maintenance of a scheme of critically unsupportable concepts and disorientating methods of setting the basic problems. In the practice of science, such a procedure is scarcely permissible. Caution is, however, called for, and unreadiness for great conceptual changes is understandable and, within certain limits, justified. The alteration of a conceptual system undoubtedly leads – at least for an interim – to difficulties of communication. But it is obvious that epistomological awareness and questioning is a pivotal requirement in a transition period such as the present. It is both a necessary enzyme and a safeguard of the current ferment's success. It is also a mode of encounter.

II MAN AS A BODILY EXISTING BEING

Undoubtedly, many linguistic aspects of a scientific transitional phase are merely temporary and provisional. This may well apply to some of the existentialist manner of speaking that is encountered at many points in this study. On the other hand, it is a significant fact about our time that it has been necessary to analyse thoroughly the conceptions of being and existing. It is significant that the verb 'to be' has achieved many new forms of usage, either forgotten ones, or ones unusual in other ways. This phenomenon is the expression of a necessary process of renewal in thinking. We had, in fact, been lapsing into a conception of being (*sein*) as almost exclusively consisting of two modes: being-usable, or being-a-concrete-object. Our continuous success through reductive controlling knowledge had begun to imply for us that it was the key to the most fundamental reality. Its conceptions had come to mean 'that which lay behind everything' for us. The mode of encounter through controlling knowledge had grown to be our only truly valid mode. It had, in fact, become the basis of all relevant experience and the criterion of its perspectives.

It is no wonder that the basic metaphysical tendency of man – to treat a part of reality as if it were the whole, with the illusion of unlimited control this contains – took this precise form in our time. The method of exact reduction has, in fact, brought man during a few centuries to a previously inconceivable mastery of nature (through technology) and human nature (primarily through medicine). The most manifold forms of destructive illness (epidemics) have been almost entirely eradicated through this method, and correction, or at least alleviation, is available for an enormous variety of complaints, defects, and disease processes.

In analysing the conception of being, the greatest contribution in our century so far has undoubtedly been made by the contemporary German thinker, Martin Heidegger. There is no space here even to begin a report on the course of his thinking or to describe his influence upon medicine, which has mainly occurred through psychiatry, and particularly through psychoanalysis and so-called psychosomatic medicine.[1] His thinking has stimulated some aspects of the analysis of bodily and organ existence presented above, and the somewhat more extended consideration that follows.

---

[1] The reader is referred to the compilation by Astrada *et al.* (1949); to the series Studies in Existentialism and Phenomenology (Tavistock Publications); and to May *et al.* (1958).

For centuries we have been fettered by a certain attitude towards our bodiliness: it is as if our primary relation to our body was that we 'owned' it, as if it 'belonged' to us only in the sense of our 'having' it. Such a separation of our body from what we are, from being-ourselves (not from our 'soul'!), led to the necessity for the basic structure discussed in Section I of this chapter: the notion of a psyche influencing a soma, and a soma influencing a psyche. If our starting-point had remained that we *are* our body (and not *merely* that we *have* a body), then a direct consequence would have followed: being-bodily-ill would have remained as one form of our being and of our behaviour (as discussed above, p. 56). But this is not what happened. On the contrary, we discovered the possibility of encountering bodiliness in terms of natural science. From this we began to experience our body as if it were possessed by the regularities, the conformity to law, we had discovered and invented. We experienced the body as an entity which had its own laws and was in some way primarily separated from ourselves as soon as 'it' stopped behaving in the way we considered obviously right and healthy and started to behave in a sick way. This also made it possible for us to experience being ill as not being sick ourselves; instead, we 'had' a disease in the body (or soul) we owned; or we were 'attacked' by it.

And the body remains fictively objective for us, as if it were primarily a disconnected and mindless – what shall we say? a machine? Thus the human meaningfulness of bodily illness has had to be interpreted with the aid of such clumsy conceptual structures as the psyche/soma solution. For instance we have tended to conceive all the processes integumented within the skin as having laws of their own: as merely pursuing certain 'natural' ends. The ends are those that happen to be the most central for the particular object of study. In connection with diseases, then, we suppose in certain cases that the psyche or psychic factors have 'got hold of' these body 'mechanisms' in some peculiar way. This mode of thinking, which has prevailed for centuries and still prevails, contains leaps and constructions that are each more remarkable than the last. One such is the tacit agreement that when a certain microscopic degree or limit is approached[1] the existence of our body will be considered to follow laws of its own. We consider that shaking hands as a greeting *is* ourselves: the handshake is part of a self-evident continuum of meaningfulness; but the behaviour of the tissues and cells in our hand is something quite different. Through such modes of conception, our organs and organ-systems have become curiously shut up inside our bodies: we do not acknowledge their presence in all our being; that is we do not realize their presence in all the multiple categories of vital relations of which our existence is composed.

We do, however, exist bodily. In a way this fact is so simple that it is complicated to speak about it. The body, our body, is a multidimensional integration. Its whole existence is a relation to something. It exists as a relation in innumerable ways: in speaking, breathing, getting food, digesting and utilizing food, excreting the waste products, being built, renewing structures, developing, adapting itself, adapting what it encounters to itself, breaking things down, becoming acquainted with the self and the not-self

---

[1] In a certain phase of the event of hearing, mechanical energy is transformed into electrical energy. The event can be characterized thus, at least. In this phase the message, as it proceeds, is 'situated' in different forms of energy, in which the hearing activity is revealed from the point of view of physics. Hardy (1965) speaks of the event of 'encoding' in hearing. But is it not true to say that it is characteristic of man in general that his existence can *always* be approached from mechanical, electrical aspects – and suchlike? And naturally one aspect proves more relevant than another depending on the goal? And is it not also true to say that in the various forms of human existence there are always hidden, concealed aspects? Sometimes concealment implies the microscopic aspect alongside or 'behind' the macroscopic aspect. At times, again, concealment implies that some concern is perhaps unconscious to the individual himself, whereas to others it is perhaps both visible and present. However, the essential thing here, it would seem, is to avoid considering without further ado that, say, the microscopic aspect, or our observation concerning electrical energy, is the most fundamental existent, and that everything else is the result or function – the caused. Is it not disorientating to think of hearing as 'the result' of the structure of the hearing organs or their electrical activity? And equally so to regard thinking, speaking, and other activities as 'cerebral functions'? It is of course true that the hearing organs function in hearing and the brain functions in thinking; but it is the man who hears and the man who thinks, not his sensory organs in a separate life of their own, although the man hears and thinks with them (as already stated above, p. 51).

and their interrelations, and so on. All the organs and organ systems are components of these existential relations: not only the respiratory, digestive, excretory, locomotive and sensory organs, for example, but the systems regulating the processes of construction and regeneration as well. In these relations the organs exist. The Latin *exsisto* means 'I stand out'. The organs exist, stand out, reach outside, beyond themselves, just as the whole organism does as an entity. (This was touched on earlier, in discussing speech.) Depending on the state of integration of the individual's various existential dimensions, his organs participate in existence. They do so in various ways and 'tuned' to various pitches and on the dimension characteristic of each organ. The hearing organism, for instance, is specifically involved in all that is heard. It is not only involved in what is listened to. It is also involved in what is not listened to, yet has a voice: what is vocally silenced because people, perhaps the majority in an 'environment', are 'deaf' to it for some reason, but which nevertheless manages to express itself. The concept of a milieu – an 'environment' – is inadequate here and may often be misleading. As bodies we do not primarily exist as separate beings, upon which various kinds of influences, such as environments and conditions, 'then' exert their effects; for our entire existence is always, from the very start, a 'being-in-relationship'.[1] Our being is, literally, a perpetual being-beyond-ourselves – an *ex-sistence*. And this, of course, concerns all our bodiliness, whether at the microscopic level or the macroscopic, inside the skin integument or outside it, healthy or sick.

Man is inconceivable without his fellow-men: to be human is to live in a community. Thus man is from the first a fellow-man. In the same way, as an 'ex-sistent', he is to begin with, and always, *in* the world, and not merely under the influence of certain environments. Since man is inherently a fellow-man and inherently 'in' the world, man *is* various particular relations, man

---

[1] If, in thought, we remove the body's 'being in relationships – to the world and itself', what remains? What we do know is that the cessation of manifest being-in-relations which is associated with death means the decomposition of the body: a radical transformation of its material mode of existence.

is interpretations of life, self, and the world, man *is* interpretations 'tuned' in a particular way. There has been much unnecessary and confusing theorization about infancy, for example, because of an initial error about a child's being: an infant has been regarded as primarily a separate and isolated being; from this premise an attempt has then been made to construct the infant's world out of the supposed 'influences' of motherhood and parenthood upon him. Yet an infant is inherently part of the human community, does not exist alone. Sexuality has been similarly isolated from its integral context. We have come to conceive of 'sex' as a kind of power or force. This misconception has occurred because we have first excluded an essential from our concept of man, from the being of man; we have ignored the fact that man *is* the man-woman relationship. Man does not 'have' sex nor is he 'driven' by it. He *is* a sexual being.[1]

III   ON THE ANTHROPOLOGY
OF SPEECH AND SOME SPEECH DISTURBANCES

Speech has a key position in the human community's processes and permanent forms of integration. It constitutes a central element in the relation of man to being in general. Without speech there would be no human history as we know it. Through speech man constructs his relation to himself, to other men, to history, to nature, and to being in general. 'Speech' here implies reciprocal comprehensibility, articulating itself conceptually; it does not mean the mere manifestation of speaking. Speech is a central and wide dimension of man's existence; and it is a basic dimension of the 'process' through which existence in its endless forms is related to man and integrated with him. (The naming of everything that exists is only one aspect of this.) Speech as an individual ability is thus only one aspect of an extensive supra-individual process and structure.

Another way of putting it would be this. Being is meaningfully present for man. Man's existence is to be in constant 'speaking

[1] Essential elements of this short analysis are contained in the writings of other authors, as, for instance, in the already mentioned Boss (1954).

relations' with whatever he encounters. In this framework, vocal or articulated speech has its own place, varying from one individual to another and according to family, social sphere, style of life, cultural milieu, and epoch. But articulated speech does not represent the whole of speech-relatedness. It can largely be replaced by other social forms of reciprocal comprehension, such as gestures, signals, braille, writing, or even pantomime. Articulated reciprocal comprehension has indeed many temporal and spatial configurations, which are distinguishable from each other. There are also mediated and immediate forms of articulated speech, and there are such techniques as recording on a magnetic tape, for example.

There are also vastly different manners of speaking. Some people *listen* more attentively than others to themselves and to their fellow-men when they are speaking. Others do not seem to have their share of time for speech: they must seize it from other people by interrupting. Others, again, cannot give their speech a clear configuration against the silence: they stumble, producing dissonant and clumsy effects of haste; and so on.

Articulated vocal speech, even including its equivalents, does not exhaust man's modes of speech relatedness. Speech relatedness is other existential modes too: it is our familiarity with and control of nature, for example; it is our possibilities of finding means of satisfying our multifarious requirements; it is our ability to construct all that we sum up as culture.

Articulated vocal speech is one central form of linguistic speech relatedness, one form of speech community. Linguistic speech community (which is not strictly distinguishable from non-linguistic forms) is an event or process, looked at from one point of view. From another point of view it is a structure, a composition, or an institution. Under its aspect as a process it includes communication: making oneself understood and becoming understood. I shall survey communication from four different points of view: A, B, C, and D.

A: Communication consists of (i) allocution and (ii) sharing. Allocution is asking, rejecting, and commanding. Sharing is the cultivation of empathy and, on the other hand, the transference of information.

B: Communication is contact with oneself and others. Communication with oneself includes thinking; it includes a listening-acquaintance with oneself – the recognition of feelings and internal images: this may extend to writing poetry or composing music. Communication with oneself also includes the sense of the self as an obligated being – usually called conscience. A sub-element of the conscience is conscience for action, or feed-back activity.

C: Speech capacity is realization of communication, or successs in the linguistic aspect of speech-relatedness. This has two basic aspects for the individual: the constitution of a speaking centre; and technical success in speaking – integrity of speech.

In the process of realizing a speech-community, human individuals are always living through each other and are dependent on each other. No generation, for instance, has entirely created the language it speaks. Clearly, too, when a child speaks, it speaks with the support of its nest – out of its nest, as it were, and through its parents; this is particularly so with speech outside the 'immediate' nest, speech to outsiders. Passing to broader fields, a nation can be said to speak through its representatives, authors, composers, and even political delegates.

Within the network of men's mutual speech relatedness, each and everyone in his special way, constitutes a speech centre. (Actually we are here dealing with the structural aspect of speech relatedness quite as much as with its process.) During the course of its evolution towards adulthood, a child may gradually come to constitute a speech centre, even a very solid one, and still have a hoarse voice, stutter, or speak nasally. In that case one technical aspect of communication may be said to be perceptibly defective or to have almost entirely failed. The statement has a validity, but it is not sufficient to describe the phenomenon. Helen Keller, who was not only severely hard-of-hearing but virtually deaf, and blind as well, came to constitute a speech centre with a high degree of differentiation and responsibility, even though she could not hear articulated speech. Failure of the technical aspect of speech communication – stuttering for example – is, I think, not merely technical: it is one of the phenomena of the process of constituting a speech centre. (No individual, let us remember, is totally free from fundamental defects, either as a speech centre or as regards technical control or 'equipment'.) I think one could validly claim, in fact, that an individual's speech defect is very far from being a technical matter alone: it is essentially a manifestation of a defectiveness in the community's speech relatedness: it belongs to certain constellations that favour the temporal and spatial focusing of the impediment on one member of the community alone.

D: How does the *process* of communication lead to a *structure* of communication? The path from process to structure is the course of development of the child's speech in two areas: in the nest, and in the reception that the community as a whole provides for the child. The reciprocal comprehension and interaction thus arising is the foundation of the structure of communication. As stated earlier, the fundamental factor for growth into communication, and for communication to be learned sufficiently for use, is a definite prerequisite: the child must be 'allowed' to be *present* to others, and the *presence* of another human being and of being in general must unfold for him. For this a nest of at least minimal stability is required, and it must be possible for the parents to be *present* for the child in some substantial way.

This prerequisite is only possible if maternity receives some protection in the marriage partnership; or, at least, if the community provides special compensatory support. Another fundamental prerequisite, among others, is that the child must receive recognition to some extent – or at least toleration for its individuality, including its defects.

We now arrive at the structural or institutional aspect of the linguistic speech community. It is general knowledge that a child's hearing and intelligence occupy central positions in speech learning. Hearing was dealt with above (pp. 51 and 105). Let us admit that hearing is more unambiguously a function than speech is. The relative autonomy of hearing is clear. It has been possible effectively to conceive of hearing from many objective, reductive controlling points of view. Not surprisingly, therefore, an almost undisturbed illusion has come to prevail: that hearing is nothing else but what it appears to be when reified in the light of reductive control; and that all the prerequisites for hearing are expressed in such information. All perception, however, is human behaviour; or, to put it more generally still, all perception is human existence: it is a mode of existing. True, perception is *relatively* independent; but nevertheless perception is integrated into an organism and dependent on it; and it is also directed towards the self, towards others, and towards the world, and 'tuned' accordingly. In all these fundamental directions, perception, including hearing, also has limits on its autonomy. The hearing organism is in imminent danger when it has would-be autonomy imposed on it: if it is asked to bear separate responsibility for hearing. The hearing is likely to break down if it is considered to bear the vicarious burden of the total organism's responsibility – if the hearing 'itself' is regarded as listening instead of the individual, the individual's stage of development, the parents or the wider community.

Intelligence, again, is a term of broad reference: its content and interpretation vary enormously from community to community and individual to individual. The concepts 'general sense' (not meaning any *special* sense, such as vision, hearing, etc.) and 'general controlling capacity' are one possible way of characterizing intelligence. Intelligence might also be defined as the capacity for mastering one's speaking relatedness with being. In this definition intelligence is intrinsically associated with linguistic speech ability, intelligence being a constituent, a structural element of speech. But this interpretation singles out man's individual *ability* to bring himself into conceptual communication. The recognition of an individual's presence in a community, however, is not exclusively dependent on his abilities. The quality and quantity of a person's inherent intellectual talents certainly impose their own limits on the person's possibilities of developing into a relatively independent speaking centre. The existence of such limits is apparent. But it is equally obvious too that the limits cannot be defined with ultimate certainty in any particular case. (These matters are also discussed on pp. 42–4 above.)

The vitality of an individual's linguistic speech relatedness is a relatively constant structure, and so is the technical success of his speech communication. Both of these are related to his potentialities. But in addition the results achieved so far, the person's developmental history, are involved too. It is not merely the cross-sectional situation that is of significance here but also the direction of progress, and whether it is possible to proceed (however modestly) on the way towards integration. We must recognize that a change in speech structure reaches deeply and extensively into the person involved, into his basic modes of existence. The kind of implication here is illustrated on pp. 63–6 above, where a case was quoted from the literature. The patient had an impediment in his speech development. Treatment led to therapeutic success, but this was followed by sudden death, raising many problems of interpretation. The preceding chapters also show that human disease can find a fertile soil in speech in innumerable ways and reach it by innumerable channels. If diseases are not explicably 'speech disturbances', then little attention is usually paid to the speech disturbance phenomena that occur in other diseases. Speech disturbance, in particular, reveals the problematic nature of the attitude that primarily attempts to eliminate the symptom. Phoniatrists and speech therapists constantly observe a reduction of hoarseness, cluttering, and stuttering, for example, within the therapeutic situation, while the patient's impediment still goes on in other situations, or recurs when the therapeutic contact is interrupted. What is involved here? Apparently we are concerned with a substitute structure of defectiveness and illness. The speech defect is a vicariousness of the sort mentioned earlier. It is not easy to give up a speech defect or disease unless the more radical problem has been faced: the individual and communal problems that have vicariously devolved on to the organs must be shared and encountered in terms of personal responsibility.

Speech is also participation in language and languages. Here too individual achievement has been stressed and documented. But clearly, the concept of speech as something contained within an individual reveals a remarkable degree of abstraction. Speech, surely, is a phenomenon that occurs primarily *between*: between a human being and himself, between one man and another, or between him and being. And since language unites men and epochs, speech is being-through-others and dependence on others. All this is something within which the individual *dwells* when he speaks. The languages that families use, the language of a tradition, the language of any composite social structure – these all contain realized interpretations of being. Through speech the individual participates in them. Language here is both a developmental dimension and a limiting factor. It is one of our most central institutionalized ways of inhabiting this world.[1] While language expresses and realizes personal, family, and national individuality, it also brings everybody into other people's spheres of influence. It also involves individuals in the supra-individual construction and process called culture. Another person's language is always simultaneously shared and alien, regardless of whether it is one's native language or the language of another nation. The recognition of each person's presence is always at stake; and so is the realization of speech between the poles of reality and appearance. The physiology and pathology of speech are (or should be)

[1] Not only different languages, but manners of speaking, too, reflect the concepts of life and attitudes to life of eras, cultural traditions, peoples, and families. Manners of speaking include not only phonetic and syntactical factors but also, for example, the occasions when one does not speak, when one speaks with particular gestures or expressions, when one speaks by acting. One must include too the order that exists in certain communal units and situations: that such and such a person naturally has the responsibility to speak, the turn to speak, and so on. Different aspects of speaking predominate in different communities. In some, informational speech is particularly cultivated; in others, self-expression has a special value; while in a third type of society speech seems to have the task of forming and creating the most central atmosphere. In some places, the aesthetic configuration of speech has an important position; elsewhere logicality of speech, understood in a certain way, is predominant; while in a third type of community the significance of the printed word is especially emphasized; and so on. All this too, of course, inevitably leaves its impression on the nature and structure of speech development difficulties and on the structure of speech impediment constellations.

concerned with all the structures outlined above.[1] This is not always easy to remember; we are often forced to limit each particular research and therapy to one partial aspect or another, even though the task relates to these structures. Yet remembering the structures is, it would seem, decisive: it is precisely such remembering that makes awakening perpetually possible. Only thus can one become sensitive to the patient's and the community's potentialities for recovery, development, and integration. Only thus can one recognize the forms of help and support available for them.

The chapter on 'Constellations' dealt with sensitivity to presence as the basis of speech, particularly when a child was learning to speak. But presence is also a whole problematic dimension where man's total relation to life and existence are concerned. Man is unsure about his fundamental presence for life. Man seriously doubts whether his presence is felt. And his way of affirming and confirming his presence for life is an overweening attempt to speak as if he knew everything already: he wants to have life summed-up and be himself the origin of all interpretations of existence. In other words he is afraid of listening to life, of being silent, of letting it unfold. He wants everything to be totalized in advance: he wants to name existence in terms of the already known. Existence is a kind of speech, but he cannot wait for the sentence to be articulated. He wants to jump ahead and finish the sentence, so that he will not be taken by surprise. Otherwise he will feel threatened, perhaps doomed.[2] Yet man also reaches out

[1] Actually, in a cross-sectional situation, the speech and hearing prerequisites for an individual's articulated speech essentially require, indeed, the intactness and good condition of certain structures and functions. On the other hand the autonomy of these structures and functions is limited: there is dependence on both the developmental history and the actual constellation in the integration process. This dependence prevails in the whole structure described above. In this respect, both destructive and constructive, or healing, networks always prevail. The process of investigation and therapy for speech and hearing impediments is bound to move in the sphere of various functions and structures: within individuals, between individuals, and in human institutions.

[2] This is an aspect of man's tendency to metaphysics, referred to several times above. Here one finds a particular application to speech and language.

to listen, and he is also inclined to be trustful. This is the other side of him, and here is a fundamental disharmony. Speech defects can be a reflection of this disharmony, and those who reflect it in their speech functions are, in a sense, more whole in their responses than those who are free from conspicuous speech defects. A person who has recourse to a speech impediment has in him, then, a healthier than usual element, even though defect and perhaps illness are the case with him too.

This seems to be clearly illustrated in the pathology of the so-called feedback function. Where speech is concerned, feedback is the individual's immediate, controlling, mostly unconscious listening (and other related proprioceptive activities) to his own speech, and the regulation of his speech in accord with these activities. In the course of the experiences of individual development, this function becomes almost autonomous and automatic. But the limited nature of this autonomy is revealed by experiences with recitation, with singing studies, and with speech disturbance, among other things. Nor are the development, structure, and functioning of feedback entirely independent of the individual's existential constellation. Would they be likely to be, in fact? Could such a controlling, listening attention to the self take place quite independently of the existential constellation? After all, in certain borderline situations (cf. above, the case of Raimo, pp. 51–2), the individual is unable to attend even to other people's speech. And in the case of Aino, for example (pp. 52–3), the child could not attend to – listen to – nest occurrences that were beyond her endurance and level of integration. Can attention, whether to the self or others, be independent of the degree of general integration?

There is good reason to assume that an individual's feedback is nuanced, in one way or another, by the relationships between the child and his world of reception. (Feedback has hardly been investigated from this point of view.) Otherwise, where could the feedback receive its background for comparison? Clearly, the background of an individual's feedback is always formed by factors that, in varying degrees, either accord with the individual's being or are alien to it. These factors result in a polarity of many different types of opposites: close–remote, stimulating–paralysing, clear–unclear, strict–lenient, remiss–vigilant, consistent–inconsistent, matter-of-fact–aggressive, flexible–rigid, tranquil–fussily insistent, and so on. Feedback is dependent on consciousness in extremely varied ways. Feedback can be repressed in different degrees. Or, in a completely split situation, feedback may have contact with only one fragment of the personality at a time. Such may be the case, for example, when there is a grave discrepancy between the voice and the personality.

Feedback is a kind of control of performance, and, as a phenomenon, it displays many features analogous to conscience. The control of performance, like the conscience as a whole, does become a constituent of the individual (with varying degrees of independence). Nevertheless, self-control, with varying degrees of sensitivity and in various ways, is in continuous communication with general standards, with other people's attitudes, and with the images formed of these. The same is true for every actual speech situation. The most varied details of speech – from flow and rhythm to tone, melody, and accentuation – undergo continuous modification due to this generality of reference. Many basic prerequisites must be fulfilled before the result is, not a speech disturbance, but a compatible adaptation to the situation.

The independence, in varying degrees, of the control of performance was referred to above.[1] In stuttering, clearly, an essential problem is dependence/independence in relation to feedback. Something fundamental in the relation between the stutterer and his community has remained unclarified, undefined: something that concerns this individual's speech control and self-control. What has happened here? Has the receiving world of the future stutterer left him in some way unacknowledged, demanded impossibilities of him, or even exerted violence towards him – in conditions in which self-expression of his essence in the speech-dimension has been a pertinent issue? In a disturbance of speech rhythm, what is involved? Is it a tactlessness in the community? However the case may be, the stutterer's self-controlling mechan-

[1] The opposite of independence is not only despairing dependency but also isolation, the feedback's separation from shared life, other people.

ism responds to a communal speech situation with stumbling and convulsions. It is as if the stutterer were at times possessed by paroxysmal suspicions that, when he speaks, something threatens him – something he must protect himself against. Apparently, too, in one side of him, he expects his fellow-men to regulate his act of speech. The case is thus one of expectation: it contains both a 'wish' and a 'fear': it relieves him of speech responsibility,[1] but on the other hand it exposes him to a danger: that this alien regulation will not occur in a way that is compatible with his essence; there even exists the possibility that he will be subjected to impossible or violent demands.

The stutterer, then, crucially locates part of his feedback responsibility in his fellow-men. He is thus especially – though most ambivalently – susceptible to alien speech rhythms. At the XIIIth Congress of the International Association of Logopedics and Phoniatrics in Vienna, 1965, during a discussion concerning the rhythmic talents of stutterers, a German logopedist adduced the case of an (adult) stutterer. The latter's treatment gradually resulted in his not stuttering during therapy situations, which is a fairly common phenomenon. However, in addition, the patient was able to speak without stuttering in other situations too, if, as suggested by his therapist, he kept a metronome running at a frequency they had agreed on.

From the psychotherapeutic point of view, this case illustrates the so-called transference cure: relief of symptoms dependent on the therapeutic relationship. This is one stage of the process of recovery. The case reflects feedback problems; it also reflects the transference and transformation process in the event of recovery, and the hiatuses.[2] Such an experience, it would seem, observably demonstrates the kind of difficulties that may be encountered by certain traditional approaches: those, namely that localize and reify the defect, regarding body-matter and the individual as the sole media of disease. For we could ask such uqestions as these.

---

[1] After the manuscript of this study was completed, I had an opportunity to read R. W. Riber's paper (1965) 'Word Magic, Self-Alienation and Stuttering'. Riber argues that self-alienation in stuttering helps the stutterer to be relieved of the responsibility for being himself in a communication situation.
[2] Cf. above, p. 77.

Where is the stuttering located? Is it in the speech organs? In the nervous tracts? In the individual's self-control? In social circumstances touching on self-control? Where was the stuttering's point of extinction in the treatment described? In the patient? In the therapist? In the metronome? And so on.

At the Vienna conference, the French logopedist Le Huche presented a method of treatment for stutterers. In this the patient has to draw any figure that comes into his mind; he must then try, through verbal instructions, to get his therapist to produce an analogous figure – without the therapist's seeing the original. After hearing this lecture, I was explaining to the lecturer my own conception of the structure of stuttering, when it emerged that he was not even acquainted with the concept of feedback. In spite of this, the method itself clearly reveals an insight into a basic element of the stutterer's feedback situation.

Cluttering or tachyphemia is, in an interesting way, a phenomenon opposite to stuttering. Cluttering too is partly a disturbance of speech rhythm, but here the flow of speech is too copious and uninterrupted. The hurried, stumbling, or otherwise unclear speech of a clutterer often does not bother the person himself at all, whereas most stutterers suffer because of their impediment. In the case of stuttering, consciousness continually seems to penetrate into what ought to be automatic; whereas for the clutterer, consciousness of the act of speaking is very dim. On the other hand, one fact is clearly common to both these types: a substantial part of the feedback responsibility has remained located in the victim's fellow-men. A stutterer's symptom is an ambivalent struggle with this dilemma, while the clutterer seems to reject the dilemma from his consciousness. If communal tactlessness is manifested in stuttering, cluttering reflects communal haste. The individual no longer undergoes this distress experientially; but when he speaks, the clutterer behaves as if he had assimilated the following conviction from his society: 'Your presence will not be felt by us unless you can jam considerably more speech than others do into any time unit. What you actually say does not interest us very much.'

Logopedic experience demonstrates that it is possible to awaken a clutterer's feedback control to a certain extent, but that it very easily relapses.

Considering the manifold dimensions, types of relations, and causes and effects in which the pathology of speech disturbance moves, we can see how rough and ready are the simplifications that are often exercised even in studies that attempt to be multi-dimensional. There is, for example, Arnold's statement concerning tachyphemia (above, p. 100). For him the organic apparently presents no problem. He also speaks about the 'linguistic function of the brain', as if this too were an equally self-evident affair. One wonders what kind of image of it he has. No doubt every reader can find a different image to fit the formula. This instance is not quoted to single out this particular scientist as uncritical, but because the case is representative. The prevailing use of language in much of the literature shows a strange inconsistency: on the one hand, it reflects an effort towards precision; on the other, it takes unexamined leaps over entirely unsolved major problems. There is a long, remarkable – and largely unexplained – 'step' from cerebral function, in the sense in which we understand it with our chemico-physico-biological concepts, to, say, speech as an act; to say nothing of speech relatedness in general. Here concepts such as 'emotional and purely pyschological causes' are allowed, by an acknowledged scientific expert, to cover the thousands of dimensions that are involved in being human in other than 'somatically' characterizable connections.

Let us here deal shortly with one dimension of the problem of cluttering. According to Arnold, who has performed extensive studies on this subject, tachyphemia is a syndrome complex: the clutterer is an individual whose speech development is retarded; his family history contains a more-than-average number of clutterers or persons with other speech disturbances; he displays dyspractic clumsiness, difficulties in right-left lateralization, unmusicalness, and a mathematical talent. To assist this syndromic angle of vision, let us adopt a method of observation that bears upon the mutual speech integration between the individual and the community. Taking the observations of Arnold into consideration, cluttering may then be seen as a developmental danger of individuals possessing certain types of talent combination: some of these persons will emerge successfully; some will develop a speech defect; while others again will be doomed to suffer from their individuality in a dimension other than speech. The outcome here may in fact depend crucially on the pressure of the communal haste referred to above. This communal haste may perhaps represent a special type of difficulty for certain types of parents. This may manifest itself as lack of patience: they cannot offer their child sufficient time for verbal expression of its individuality. This haste may, then, be the narrow gate for such an individual.

It may well be that the outline just presented misses the mark in some details. The point here, however, is one of principle: the way of thinking. The notion that a certain combination of talents in itself is to blame for a speech impediment, such as cluttering, obviously contains a simplication. And, from a practical point of view, the notion can be crucially disorientating.

CHAPTER 5

The Disease Process

I HOPE, DESPAIR, AND THE HISTORY OF RECEIVING: THE FORMATION OF THE DISEASE (DEFECT) PROCESS

This chapter will take up certain points that have already received a preliminary treatment. First, let us return to the statement that a disease process always takes the form of a challenge – and a response, the way the challenge is received. There is no such thing as disease 'in itself': disease does not present itself objectively for scrutiny as a given, non-equivocal phenomenon. Disease 'in itself' can only be found in abstractions serving quite special and narrowly limited purposes.

In disturbances of speech development, the disease process often consists of a defect and its reception. My earlier analysis has shown, however, that the defect itself originated as part of the history of reception. It appeared in the course of certain events: pregnancy, the formation of gametes, the choice of partner, and so on. Very often the 'defect' is actually a natural variation. But in a certain type of society and in a particular time, when for example a narrow concept of 'reality' prevails – reality considered as knowledge already possessed and reified – each manifestation of the variation is experienced discriminatorily: it is seized on as a defect.[1]

Then of course there are 'transitions' from constellations like this to ones displaying manifold and manifest deficiencies. But

---

[1] For comparison, many Syrians consider the Egyptians are doomed, for, in the opinion of these Syrians, the Egyptian palate is arched in a way that makes it impossible for them ever to learn to pronounce the name Allah properly.

even when defectiveness is at its most conspicuous, the following is a decisive factor. How far are the deficiencies recognized and acknowledged as communal? And how far, on the other hand, is the bearer of the defect branded as an 'outsider', or as having 'a special and isolated fate'. If the individual is thus branded and then despair takes hold of the branded individual as well, as a hidden structure, the morbid advance of the destructive process is already well-prepared.

Human life, community life, is so structured that a defect does not, as such, and without more ado, imply misfortune or impoverishment for the individual or the community. Nor does it from the point of view of the defective person's self-recognition, his experience of himself, and his suffering of himself – from the point of view of his 'happiness', therefore. A defect, as such, does not imply determination in any direction. The individual's happiness is in the continuous unfolding of his experience, and also in the fruitfulness of his suffering. The criterion of his happiness is his power and permission to grow into his own self, with all that this involves. This, in turn, depends on other circumstances: the reality or mere ostensibility of his reception; the degree to which he is allowed, together with his defects and inherited birth constellations, to become integrated into his community; and the degree to which the community is permitted to become integrated into what he, the individual, represents. A defective fate, then, is structured in terms of the reflectivity between the self and the community. An individual's defect is entwined in the texture of history, both the individual's and the community's. The defect constitutes an unpaid debt to life. The defect contains a hidden and undeveloped potentiality, needing expression, demanded by life as a debt, a return for the offer of life. Life demands life. As a debt to life, the defect thus constitutes a challenge – to search for a way through the defect to the 'hidden treasure' that underlies it. What looks like a debt on the surface turns out to be a cache of treasure, of 'unlived life', awaiting unfoldment and development. The defect is an invitation to discover the individual and communal potentialities that have so far remained unlived, locked up and concealed in the defect constellation. Sometimes the reverse side of the defect contains more than an ordinary undeveloped potentiality: an interesting special talent may inhere in it, now manifesting as a defect. Sometimes, too, the defect draws special attention to some potentiality that would otherwise be overlooked, and leads to its cultivation. The potentiality discovered and developed may be in the individual or in the environmental community, or in both.

As such, then, a defect does not always imply direct unhappiness, although a defect is always an affliction. The way we relate ourselves to the history of origin of the defect profoundly affects the form the defect takes as a 'fate' of both the individual and the community: this even includes the form the disease process will take. The truth of this is surely obvious, if only because effective analysis of certain causative aspects of the defect may give us the possibility of correcting or compensating for the defect to some extent. At the same time, however, there is another circumstance. Our attitudes towards the history of origin of the defect modify the continuous influence of the defect's causal network upon the formation of the disease constellation. This remains true even if the causes no longer induce visible and perceptible new damage to the organs. Let us consider Raimo's case, for example (pp. 51–2). The kind of relationship the boy develops to his defective hearing will most certainly depend on something supra-individual, something communal. It will depend on how far the aspect of the family constellation that originally proved destructive to Raimo can become the productive responsibility of his parents. It will depend, that is, on how far the parents awaken to the destructive aspect of the constellation and are able to share in the process of improvement. This family constellation did, after all, contribute to the origin of the hearing defect. Since it did so, we cannot predict how any changes in a continuously influential causal network might eventually manifest, say, in the subsequent condition of the acoustic organ. But one thing is certain. These changes will be felt: they will be felt, for example, in how the patient learns to hear within the framework that is provided by the functional possibilities of his hearing organs. This again will affect his learning to speak, and so on.

Naturally, defects in the prerequisites for learning and commanding speech, of whatever kind, demand a specially favourable
constellation, if the remaining potentialities are to be effectively
activated: if, that is, the patient is to be allowed to constitute a
speech centre in a way that is natural to him. Such an optimal
situation is very rarely given. In most cases it is only attainable, if
at all, through prolonged therapeutic work within the framework
of a team. The reception of defectiveness and the integrative
growth of a defective individual into the community as a whole
are always problematic and difficult; often a rather complete
failure ensues. Nor is this to be wondered at when one remem-
bers another fact: often we may see, more or less clearly, or
perhaps only suspect, that the origin of the defect is connected
with the basic attitudes of the very communities, the entities, into
which integration needs to take place. The history of reception
of the defect is also presented as simply a continuance of the
history of origin of the defect: the reception tends to maintain its
initially destructive direction. The desire to be distanced, removed
from the defectiveness in ourselves and in others – to get rid of
it – is the motivation for a reduced, limited and one-sided encounter with the defect constellation: one restricts one's view to
distinctly isolated parts and aspects of it. The specific form that
the disease process takes also depends particularly on the type of
participation of those who have encountered the problem in
themselves and others. 'Decisions' must be made at every step,
and these decisions that the participants make shape the process.
Despair and discrimination, in their many guises, constitute
dimensions in the process of disturbance and speech development.
From moment to moment, and from place to place, the direction
of the process will be determined – even 'decided' – by the extent
to which the people that the challenge is reaching can identify
their own despair and discriminatory attitudes, by how far they
dare to struggle with these. Such identification, again, is only
possible if there is hope; and hope cannot be patented, only
cherished. In encounters with disease, then, one important basic
dimension of the struggle is how reception will proceed in the
future. Will the future history of reception continue along the

same lines as before? Or will the history of reception gradually be transformed? Will there be a new process in the patient and the people now surrounding him?

II DISEASE AS AN ALARM, AND THE TRANSFERENCE AS THE ALARM RECEIVED

A disease process is constantly eloquent in some way: it is sounding an alarm, or at least giving a reminder, concerning an aspect of life that is threatened by distortion or suffocation. Wherever an individual's presence is not sufficiently realized, either for himself, or his fellow-men, something of an appeal always takes its place. 'Life takes care' of that. Disease's reminder is both potent, in very different ways and degrees, and veiled. This enveilment is clearly not a separate property of the symptom. Its degree depends on, is a function of, the ambivalent receptivity of the community to the individual potentiality for life contained in the symptom. The ambivalence is twofold. First, the individual potentiality is both burying itself in the symptom and sounding the alarm through the symptom. And secondly, both the individual and the community are simultaneously closed and open to the message of the buried potentiality. Clearly, the symptom becomes increasingly remote as an appeal, the more its message is ignored; at the same time it becomes more massive from the point of view of the individual. Its quality as an address is progressively lost as hope diminishes.[1] (The connotations of 'hope', here, are complex: they include hope that a sense of common responsibility for the dilemma will be awakened; hope that personal responsibility will be restored; hope of relieving the

[1] This phenomenon has been described by Viktor von Weizsäcker and by his pupils, particularly Kütemeyer (1963). They performed numerous analyses of their internal medical patients. Boss (1954) has also lucidly described the transference of bodily symptoms from one level to another: the direction was towards an increasing humanly articulated presence, an address which finally became more obvious to all. The development occurred in the course of psychoanalytic therapeutic processes. The treatment offered the patients certain elements of listening-reception, such as they had largely lacked previously. My paper 'Schizophrenia: A Human Situation' (1963) describes a radical transformation of the challenging symptom in a patient with Parkinson's disease.

diseased organ of a burden that does not belong to it; hope of growth.)

Both the negative and the positive developments proceed through transferences and transformations of the symptom. Rejection, suppression, and silencing of the message do so; and so do new vitality, liberation, and integration – 'recovery', that is. The whole community is involved in the chain of transference and transformation in either direction. The more radical the failure of reception is (as for the Kaspar children) the more the community will be penetrated by the event and its consequences. The damage will go deeper and wider. In such a case the transference of symptoms might follow some such pattern as this. The symptom will pass from speech impairment to the intestinal tract; from there to the skin; from the skin to the lungs; from the lungs to psychotic or psychopathic behaviour (in contrast to previously calm but shallow interpersonal relations). The next step may be repression of fear, or escape-reactions, among the family members or the therapeutic personnel; then there may be crises of the entire therapeutic institution; stands may be taken by adjacent organs in the community; and so on. Which transference constituted the 'first' one is naturally always relative in nature, for the chain always continues indefinitely into the past. Let us, however, make our starting-point the reception of the individual in question. In other words, we shall start from the imposition of a community problem on a particular person. A difficulty that is properly a communal responsibility is imposed on the whole organism, or on a particular organ, of an emerging and evolving individual – one who, as yet, has not actually been composed into an individual.

The community now has an opportunity – through its therapeutic team. Is the community prepared to accept this opportunity? Can it at least sound the possibility of taking its share of the responsibility? If so – if and when it thus begins to listen – the move will lead to another transfer or transference. 'Transference' indicates the gradual transmission of the problem until it becomes a joint-responsibility of the receiving part of the community, which in this case is the therapeutic team, now sharing the problem with the patient. (Hitherto only this *second* transfer has been generally and consciously regarded as 'transference', but the problem was already *transferred* on to the patient.)

This accepted form of 'transference' makes it possible for a symptom to become transformed in a new direction: progress may now occur towards an increasingly human manifestation of the underlying dilemma: there may be a move towards articulation of the dilemma in the community. If so, a third transfer is then possible: individuals or groups of people may gradually begin to appropriate their own share of responsibility. In doing so they are actually appropriating their own individual potentialities for living, making them their own, and accepting their own historical situation as a continuing personal battlefield.

This becomes possible for the following reason. Hitherto they have had to live under the distorting and burdening influence of a denied problem. But now this problem is coming within the sphere of common responsibility, and in doing so it is changing its configuration and gradually assuming human features. It is thus coming within the scope of human measures. The team's commonly gained insight, which has grown up during examination and treatment, is a new situation: an encounter between the dilemma and the sense of communal responsibility, an interpenetration of the two. This is a penetration into the disease constellation's hiatuses of transmission and transformation. It is a revelation of the meshes of the causal network in a broader human sense. The new situation thus implies a reversal of the absoluteness of the first transfer. And it may lead, through transference, to the third transfer: a new integration.[1]

[1] Within the framework of Sonninen's team, too, we have experienced how the challenges of the disease constellations make it necessary to re-evaluate one's own participation in the elements of the community's 'first transfer'. The course of the symptom's transformation, as outlined above, was thus felt in the team in many ways. The process of improvement – a profound transformation – appeared to us as an upsetting of many balances; it was only rarely a 'nice' occurrence. The fates of Pentti and Heikki are eloquent evidence of this.

CHAPTER 6

Prognosis

I DIMENSIONS OF PROGNOSIS

These, then, are factors significant for the formation of the prognosis: the openness and dynamic nature of the team, and the team's resources of endurance.[1] For the team are a community of people who have undertaken the therapeutic reception and have their own constellation, with its own inherent potentialities.

But before we go on to analyse the manifold factors affecting the prognosis in constellations with disturbance of speech development, we must consider something else. What is prognosis actually concerned with in these contexts? What is the prognosis *for*? Immediately, we see that a deficiency of articulated speech is specifically limited to the speech capacity in only very few cases – and is certainly not so limited in severe cases. The practical problem is different where mild difficulties of pronunciation and use of the voice are concerned. But in more severe cases, like those in the present study and Sonninen's paper, for example, defectiveness of articulated speech is almost invariably an aspect of a wider constellation of defectiveness in abilities and control. And this constellation in turn is part of a still wider disease constellation. At times an autistic psychosis can be established;

---

[1] Essential factors here include the relations of the therapeutic unit to the wider community that has granted the team authorization: for instance, the relation of the ward to the department; the relation of the department to the medical direction of the hospital; the mode of relatedness of the entire hospital system to the community, etc.

at others a psychopathy; at others again oligophrenia; or a considerable defect in hearing; or severe deformity of the appearance and/or organs of articulation; or weakness of perception and control associated with defectiveness of the organ responsible for general sense and general control (the brain); all these either separately or in different combinations. And here the speech impairment (in the more special sense) may form a significant partial problem, varying in degree and kind. Thus, from traditional medical points of view as well, an impediment in speech development is primarily a symptom of the most varied defects and diseases. I have attempted to show that these defects and diseases, in their turn, are parts of wider constellations, whose phenomenologies – and thus their systematics as well – are only gradually taking form.

In so far as a speech impediment implies the rupture of reciprocal social comprehensibility, its correction is of decisive significance for both the individual and the total development of the situation. The learning of articulated speech is not, however, always possible, whereas other ways of speaking *can* be achieved. The fundamental question here is establishment of the presence: the presence of the patient to others; the presence of others to the patient; and the presence of the patient to himself. For a child, the primary concern is the situation between him and his parents. Actually, the significance of learning to speak varies enormously, in both value and nature, according to the situation. For an autistic child, learning to speak offers new possibilities of contacts – with people other than his parents, with whom contacts have proved crucially fruitless. This is tremendously important for an autistic child; but, in addition, the event of learning, as such, means a rupture of the circle of despair for such a child: he may now realize that non-communication with the parents does not necessarily mean that there are no other possibilities of contact. For an oligophrenic, learning to speak can mean the discovery of new possibilities of self-expression and self-esteem, as well as a far wider possibility of utilizing his own developmental resources. On the other hand, it may also be an extra burden – the burden of having to please the teacher and others who are demanding speech. The technical learning of correct speech may be extremely testing where speech impairment is a central alarm concerning some severely distorted family constellation. And in a child with a cleft palate and nasal speech, learning to speak more naturally may reduce the weight of discrimination resting on him, though here it is at least equally important for the attitudes of the people in the closer and wider communities to develop.

Clearly, then, it is not easy to reach a general formula that would reveal what a prognosis is concerned with in any particular case. Cases can apparently only be classified, as regards prognosis, for quite specific stages and levels of the encounter. Moreover, every constellation seems ultimately to require its own specific scale. The prognosis must be determined step by step according to the specific scale. But, of course, the prognosis naturally has some relatively unambiguous aspects as well. Can the fault be totally eradicated, or not, through certain measures? Can it be corrected, or not? If it can, to what extent? Can effective means of compensation be developed for the defect? Is the delay in speech development of the sort that is usually made up in a few years, without any special treatment? Relevant preventive, corrective and eradicative measures for defects include the avoidance of a rubeola infection during pregnancy; or the removal of a rubeola-damaged foetus from the uterus (terminating the growth); Rh-control; prophylaxis against brain injury during deliveries; the prevention of premature ossification of symphyses between the cranial bones; interventions preventing the development of hydrocephalus; diet for a child with phenylketonuria; cleft palate operations; surgical procedures for correcting deformation of the hearing organs; the use of a hearing aid by hard-of-hearing people; and so on. Lip-reading is an example of compensation; so is sign language. Here another question arises. How far have children who are relatively free from speech impairments – the so-called healthy children – been educated and encouraged to accustom themselves to including people with sensory defects within their sphere of communication, when necessary? This is clearly one of the most elementary possibilities of provid-

PROGNOSIS

ing compensation for defects. It is an ever-present factor affecting the prognosis.

If the question of prognosis is presented simply, it can often also be answered fairly readily. Does this child possess enough general ability to learn articulated speech? Sometimes, again, the degree of cerebral injury is so grave that permanent limitations on learning are undoubtedly imposed.

In any case, however great or small the possibility of correction, the problem always involves mutual integration between the patient and his several communities. Even if no obvious defect is left to burden him, or the defect has been decisively decreased, the constellation in which the defect arose may still exert an inhibiting influence upon the process of reintegration. And this can be so even if the correction or compensation of the defect has been very successful. It can be so even if reintegration has already occurred to some extent. The degree of correction of the fault, therefore, does not exclusively decide the total success of the reintegration. Thus, there are good reasons for asking whether a natural goal of healing would not be this: a living integration process in motion. This, rather than the isolated disappearance of the defect – imagined as an event that can be clearly defined in advance – is a perhaps more productive aim. The prognosis, one might argue, is essentially concerned with the discovery of a way to mutual integration. Prognosis concerning the technical defects merely constitute partial factors of this total prognosis. Here again the pertinent question is not merely the probability or improbability of attaining a certain level of obvious integration. The question is rather to study where the possibilities will be found for a starting point – towards integration, and away from chaos and destruction.

The question in prognosis, then, is not whether there is hope or not, or to what degree. On the contrary, it might be said that hope is a prerequisite for relevant prognostication. Hope, indeed, reaches towards integration. Hope is continued belief (in spite of everything) in the existence of a healing communal integration underlying the factually experienced disease and dismemberment: unifying tendencies exist in the very spot where a disintegrating

131

community is about to forget its organismic nature.[1] Hope thus includes, among other things, the belief that no irreversibility encountered by us amounts to the feared and hidden spectre of death itself.

In all the disease constellations encountered, the struggle for improvement is already going on, and participation in this struggle is always indicated. The disease itself, for its part, is also an expression of the organism's ability to sound the alarm, to respond to some destructive constellation, implying chaos, disorder. And an alarm is an invitation to participate in the battle for improvement, even though, from a certain point of view, the battle may initially seem to be a losing one. The essence of disease includes this: the persons involved in the disease constellations offer the invitation ambivalently: they appeal for both improvement and the maintenance of the status quo; indirectly they may even appeal for destruction. In answering this summons, one is thus forced to estimate the resistances to improvement – where they lie, what kind they are, how strong, which way they are moving, how fast, and on what fronts. Only thus can one obtain the most appropriate strategy for each advance, taking into account the properties of the team.

II FACTORS AFFECTING PROGNOSIS

The team, which estimates the prognosis, is both a participant in the battle and the battlefield itself. In every case, the persistence of the team is one aspect of the stability of the therapeutic constellation, and it undoubtedly has a central significance for the prognosis. This stability is also dependent on many other things. For example, how integrated is the country's medical service? It can be very relevant to the patient, for instance, whether he lives in a remote district or in some larger centre of population. Poverty of the family can also be an obstacle to mobility. Ignorance, or backwardness of other sorts, in the area of residence may create serious difficulties. Many so-called 'conditions' are involved here. These conditions always seem to include some attitude of

[1] Cf. A. Siirala (1964).

the people involved in the constellation. Moreover, the 'conditions' may contain manifest or disguised community discriminations, or other attitudes of despair. A dominating factor of prognosis is the discovery of a responsible centre – some family member, or other person strategically significant for the patient, who is ready to take responsibility in a relatively productive way. The amenableness to treatment of the members of the child's nest, primarily the mother and father, is important: the smaller, or more helpless developmentally, the child is, the more essential this amenableness is. Again, a much rougher prognostic factor is the general coherence or incoherence of the family: whether the child is an orphan; extreme disharmony between the parents, or separation; mental disease in either of the parents; alcoholism; criminality; or radical family poverty. Modern society is, however, increasingly assuming responsibility for such situations: through welfare measures and institutions, for instance, in accordance with its legislation for the protection of children.

On the other hand, no legislation can guarantee the vitality of the struggle for care. Vitality too is decisive in each family constellation, no matter how miserable the framework. Is the family congealed in its relations within itself and with the larger community outside? Or does the family move productively in some dimension? The family's situation concerning speech is naturally a most essential factor for the development of the child's speech. A gross discrepancy between what is said and the atmosphere that vibrates wordlessly will affect the foundations of speech. Lack of mutual respect and failure to acknowledge personal boundaries can be crucially felt in the feedback development. And so can the general hastiness and tactlessness associated with domination. Scantiness of speech, sheer quantitative meagreness of speech, or a family's general isolation, or an atmosphere of suspicion in the home – all these are apt to prevent the development of wider surfaces of contact with the community: they interfere with the dialogue outwards.

The constellation of prognosis can also be moulded by many other factors. A list would include the following: the lack of music, or the distortion of it; the father's, or mother's, voice monopolizing the vocal space; radio or television perpetually on, permitting some family member to tyrannize over the others; defects of speech in other family members, and the parents' attitude towards these; indifference; resignation; feelings of shame in front of others; a perfectionistic compulsion to rectify even the slightest deviations from the parents' speech ideals; and so on. And of course, in particular, the parents' attitude towards the patient's speech defect has a special prognostic significance.

Here, then, we come to the significance that the speech impairment has in the patient's personality dynamics, in his family's dynamics and in the dynamics of the other pertinent social groups. These are all factors that influence the prognosis. What significance does the speech impediment have for our patient's social performance and achievements? And how does he feel and vitally experience the impediment – in so far as such experiencing has become part of the child, as its own felt perception? What is the estimated influence of the speech impairment on the child's general possibilities of development? To what extent do the parents see the defectiveness of their child or comprehend its nature? And to what extent have they awakened to responsibility for seeking help? How far can the parents be motivated towards participating in the disentanglement? Often the existence of a defect is not acknowledged at all. At times, again, an overprotective, overconcerned, pitying and perhaps suffocatingly compensatory attitude prevails in the parents, depriving the child of many of his incentives towards speech.

Quite often, again, what is encountered is a rigidly violent attempt to have the disturbance eradicated, once and for all, through commands and constant advice. As already pointed out in this study, sometimes the impediment moves the parents to reject, even abandon, the defective child. Naturally, it is crucial for the child if they can hardly bear to acknowledge him as their own in the face of the community. Of course, one can list weighty prognostic factors in the other direction: recognition of the child as their own, with all his defects; a sensitive eye and ear for the child's individuality and the residual potentialities of the defective aspect; loyalty and patience; and imaginative initiative concerning the child with a speech defect. These, however, are only possible when the parents have a similarly lively, hopeful and tolerant relation to themselves. And such an attitude requires successful liberation from certain communal tendencies: attitudes that have been dealt with above in various ways, such as our tendencies to use discriminatory practices as a way of localizing the death we fear. In the case of speech impediments, such discriminatory practices specifically and directly increase and distort the defects. The apprehension felt by a person who is rejected, perhaps latently persecuted, multiplies his speech difficulties. On the other hand, again, open receptiveness, patience, and interest in securing the patient's participation in the communal life, and his personal contribution, lead to the discovery of apparently non-existent resources. They can even make a child function with destroyed resources, as we saw in the case of the aphasic child described in the chapter 'Aetiology'.

Particularly with children who have especially great defects or wide disablements, the discovery and mobilization of their remaining resources are potent in significance. And this does not apply to speech resources alone. It shows what elementary significance it has for a human being to have his individuality acknowledged in the very presence of his defects and the distortions and involvements of his receptional history. Of course, the prognosis for the correction of the technical aspect of the defect also depends on the general intelligence and good early developmental history of the child. But the principal goal must still be communal and joint integration of what is encountered in the constellation and can be brought to light, however defective and unattractive this may turn out to be in some of its aspects.

The ward observation notes in the case records revealed such observations as the following about the gifts and inclinations of children with speech impairment. 'The patient is gay, energetic, loyal, generous, has bodily strength, is agile, dexterous, lively, active, can act on his own, and his power of observation is good.' 'The child shows a good capacity for recollection in this or that respect (although the power was apparently poor on the whole);

he has such and such a verbal ability, a sense of rhythm, and/or some other kind of musical talent, some vocal gifts, the ability for manifold communication through facial and other gestures, or tones of voice, an ability to mimic the cries of animals or other children's ways of speech, an ability to express himself in drawing or painting, a good ability for arithmetic, a zeal for learning and persistence in training, a good capacity for concentration, personal initiative, and so on.'

Let us take as an example eight-year-old Simo, who suffered kernicterus soon after birth, due to Rh-incompatibility. His movements were athetotic, and in particular the articulation was very elementary: there was dyslalia mechanica et functionalis, dysarthria. The same boy was found to be able to ride a bicycle quite well, was especially skilful at building with blocks, and was quite a talented little actor. Thus he had remarkable specific talents and abilities to compensate for his affliction.

The older the child, the greater is the prognostic significance of his own relation to his defectiveness. How far can the child recognize his own defectiveness and allow an adult to aid and support him in his process of integration? Can the child accept a hearing device? The compatibility of hearing devices is a very delicate matter and forms a characteristic associated problem. Can the child, in his troublesome task of integration, be patient with the adults' unawareness, their failure of intuition and their frequent wounding tactlessness? If so, this is a favourable prognostic factor. The so-called social abilities and gifts have their own prognostic value: thus adaptation to ward life and the ward children's communal games is a useful talent, if associated with a capacity for refusal and defiance when necessary. Social ability sometimes flashes up surprisingly, even in a Kaspar-child that has recently arrived in the ward: the very child who usually treats other children sadistically can, in certain situations, hurry to protect and assist helpless ones who have landed in distress.

Four-year-old Onni belonged to the Kaspars, the severely neglected children. He was born prematurely at the end of his mother's series of frequent deliveries. The parents in the family – amidst distress – spent very little time with the children in general.

At the age of one-and-a-half Onni suffered encephalitis. While in the ward, the boy developed conspicuously and learned speech eagerly from what he heard. But then he also had special gifts of charm and ability for contact: observational notes made during ward therapy included such remarks as 'marvellous eyes', and 'an ability to surpass his normal performances considerably when contact is obtained'.

Vesa has already been referred to (p. 87). He was an orphanage boy, prematurely born, and intellectually poorly gifted. It was noted in the ward that he 'brightened from his apathy', and that 'the boy who had given an impression of being passive was capable of personal initiative and also natural opposition'. He also proved eager to take care of younger children.

Perhaps we should consider here specific factors affecting prognosis negatively. For instance, quite special weaknesses could be observed in Vesa and in his constellation: he proved immature, with no power of concentration, and he had a short attention span. Perhaps the weightiest factor, here, however, was that neither of the child's parents – he was illegitimate – maintained any kind of contact with him. As regards his need for parents and to experience the related emotions of a child for father and mother, Vesa was thus entirely dependent on the contacts in the orphanage. Again, severe physical deformities or, perhaps, nasal speech imply an unfavourable prognosis, as the intolerance of the community may create friction. An especially severe therapeutic starting-point is the threat of repeated separation for a Kaspar child, though this is in another kind of dimension. Such a situation occurred for Pentti and Heikki. They were originally in a Kaspar situation, but an intensive process of contact had been set in motion through the devotion of the team to these children, and their expenditure of time and intensity. But then, for various reasons, this therapeutic constellation was broken: the child lost the persons who, through their mode of being present for him in his environment, constituted promises of emerging closeness. It is very hard to induce a child who has been subjected to torture like this to surrender himself once again to a new risk of disappointment in a subsequent close therapeutic relationship. This, then, is a prognostic factor that is structured in the vicissitudes that occur to a therapeutic community. Or, from the patient's point of view, the prognostic factor is in the phases of his therapy.

The process of contact is often at its greatest density in play therapy. Play therapy, as is well known, is the cultivation of therapeutic communication between two people, a trained psychotherapist and a child, as a developmental process. In play therapy difficulties and potentialities of the constellation are lived through. In this process they are rediscovered so that they can be integrated in and for the child. How much realization occurs in play therapy at any particular time is, of course, not independent of the total therapeutic constellation. In play therapy, however, the total therapeutic process often reaches its culmination, and frequently (not always) it is just here that the deepest distress and the most real progress become manifest. In that sense this form of therapy has a special position with regard to prognosis. In it the phases of emergence of mutual presence – the basic motive for speech – are often felt dramatically.

Sometimes a child's grasp of his play therapy is so firm that he manages to bring in all the persons involved in the constellation, even his reluctant family circle. Erik, for instance, manifested this sort of ability for vital and persistent concern for himself. He was capable of intensive participation in his own therapy, provided he was 'merely' given a therapeutic framework and a partner in the play therapy. Such an ability in a child can be regarded as part of the wealth of his personality. And this resource is so clear a prognostic factor that it is underlining the obvious to point out that it should be included in a survey or list of prognostic factors.

Finally, the simplest way of putting the matter is perhaps this. There are, in fact, a number of constellations – ones containing, for instance, autistic psychoses and neurotic or otherwise gravely disturbed behaviour – which often come up for medical treatment as, more or less simply, speech development disturbances, for that is how they are primarily experienced. That this should be the case is not greatly to be wondered at, after all. Let us only consider how extensively, at certain ages of the child, speech represents him and his general development. The child is his speech.

III PROGNOSIS, EXPERIENCE
OF THE ACTUAL SITUATION, AND EVALUATION

Cross-sectional studies of capacities for performance – that is, the various tests and other measurements – have their own essential, though only roughly, orientative value. Their significance is certainly enhanced if they are studied in the light of the experiences gained of the constellation – extended observations obtained over long periods. They can also be illuminated by anamnestic data. In this manner a picture can be obtained that is even prognostically relevant. It may concern, for example, the level of the patient's capacities for experiencing and general control. Other relevant data would concern the condition of his various capacities for performance: what his powers of visual and auditory discrimination are, for example; how far he can control statics and motility; and the condition of various forms of co-ordination. One must have more than a clear picture of degrees of ability and disturbance. One must also know the direction in which the various elements of the situation are moving. Sometimes an annually performed test may, for example, show that the patient reveals retarded development; but it may show, too, that continuous progress is occurring. Sometimes, too, it becomes clear that a destructive organic process is present and progressive. A corrective manipulatory measure may then, perhaps, be called for and feasible. But all this must be accompanied by sensitive listening. One must not lose one's alertness for a possible concealed and unheard alarm-signal in the total situation. The disentanglement may need a totally new orientation. The tests may help, but they will not reveal one 'automatically'.

A child's standing as regards speech is delineated in the observations that the phoniatrist makes during repeated examinations. His speech attainments are also indicated in the experiences with the logopedist during speech therapy sessions. But the child's speech attainments are also felt in play therapy and everyday life in the ward; that is in the patient's contacts with the nurses, the kindergarten teacher, the nurse-maids, and the other children. The significance of his forms of verbal behaviour, of the variations in degree of performance, and of the phases in general can, however, only be grasped through comprehension of what the therapy is as a total event, and this can only be obtained through sharing the experiences of the various departmental members of the team.

The decisive element in analysing the nature of a hearing impediment may be acquaintance with the child obtained over a prolonged period in the ward. All in all, a sufficiently protracted encounter with the child on a wide enough plane is necessary for elucidation of his state of communication. As regards prognosis, it is important to establish the status of his speech in a situation that is as natural for the child as possible. Similarly, it is essential to observe changes in the status of his speech that depend on the situations in various areas of the ward life. Short moments of encounter in the ward between the patient and his relatives can be particularly illuminating.[1] Questions such as the following must be continually under consideration. What is the position of speech and comprehension of speech in this child's total communication? To what extent does the child resort to sign language, and how successfully can he thereby establish the contact he wants? What kinds of things receive verbal expression? To what types of people and in what kinds of situation does the child speak? What stops or disorganizes the child's speech? What kind of vocabulary does he have, both as regards extent and in relation to his most obvious needs and wants? To what extent does the tone of the child's voice function as a mediator of message? The process implicit in these questions is often reflected with surprising clarity in the course of the multidimensional day. In the ward it is also possible to obtain a view of how and to what degree the patient responds to the challenges that are natural to a child of his age. Gradually, too, one can comprehend the extent to which his receiving world is, as a whole,

[1] See, for example, the case of Lauri (above, p. 26).

significantly present to him and alluring him towards real speech. The text at this point could actually be read as a discussion of diagnostics as much as prognostics. Indeed, in a phoniatric ward and out-patient department working on a rather long-term schedule, diagnostics and prognostics do almost merge. The first rough classification for selecting the patients in need of more extensive investigation and more thorough therapy is closer, in fact, to the traditional nature of diagnostics.

Sometimes there has hardly been time to start elucidation of the case before resistances accumulate. Sometimes too these resistances assume the form of the most commonplace impediments, apparently having nothing specifically to do with 'the disease itself'. It is impossible to get a telephone connection; letters to local welfare officials are not answered in time; some member of the team repeatedly forgets to perform an important practical task; and so on. This kind of indefinable 'initial muddle' may be a symptom of a particularly extensive and profoundly destructive constellation, determined by the most diversified factors. Sometimes, again, the 'initial muddle' rapidly yields to the continued efforts of the team. How the therapeutic disentanglement goes forward, and how far it manages to continue, understandably have a far-reaching prognostic significance. Sometimes some element in the child's situation mobilizes some resistance among the team, one that cannot be overcome, because the team cannot bear to identify it and pool their joint forces to meet it. Persistent incompatibility in the team – an incapacity for a productive interchange and mutual settlement, for difference without a rupture of the basic unanimity – will have disastrous results for many patients. Further, a persistent allergy to certain types of problems and to certain degrees of tension often prevails among teams. Truncation of the disentanglement is particularly disastrous if the team leaves the persons involved with the impression that the elucidation was pursued as far as was feasible. On the other hand, there are surprising therapeutic reversals: a problem has ended, from the team's perspective, in the gloomiest of constellations and in therapeutic impotence: and yet a clarification occurs elsewhere along channels that may be heard about much later. This may take place even when a family interrupts treatment and removes the child from therapy. What may have happened is that a fertile seed of unrest has been sown, in spite of everything, and it germinates later in some subsequent, more favourable, constellation.

CHAPTER 7

Examination and Treatment

I A DIALECTIC BETWEEN REDUCTIVE
CONTROL AND JOINTLY RESPONSIBLE AWARENESS

The word 'examination'[1] can have two connotations: (i) tests
performed on a patient, and (ii) scientific research on illness.
Scientific research can comprise all systematic acquisition of
knowledge about disturbances of speech development. Its sphere
includes treatment, examination of the patient and many other
concerns. The account of constellations in the earlier chapters of
this book should show one thing very clearly: the more extensively a defect or disease affects the total personality of man as an
organism, the more all forms of examination, investigation, and
research on the patient constitute part of the therapy. This of
course includes investigatory exchanges with the family. Contrariwise, there are numerous matters which can only be discovered and clarified through treatment, and during it. In most
cases, a substantial improvement, in some dimension at least,
seems to be a precondition for acquiring an essential total view
of the genesis and structure of the disease. Only on that basis is it
possible to obtain reliable information concerning the constellation originally encountered by the therapeutic team. Viktor von
Weizsäcker has written extensively of the interinvolvement of
examination, research, and treatment where internal medical

[1] The distinction here more particularly concerns the connotations of the Finnish
word *tutkimus*, which is translated as 'examination', 'investigation', or 'research',
depending on the context. The word 'examination' does, however, have the two
connotations in English too.

diseases are concerned. Moreover, psychoanalysis, throughout its entire history, illustrates how a therapeutic method is simultaneously an instrument of examination and research. On the other hand, however, psychoanalytic therapy has highlighted another experience: if one aims to collect and store information in the course of the therapy itself, this may make it difficult or even impossible to secure the desired information:[1] one's attitude makes the harvest trivial, and the level of therapy declines. In some sense this finding probably has a bearing on all the interrelations between a relatively holistic therapy and attempts to gain knowledge. Sympathetic awareness, devotion, openness, and, on the other hand, systematic efforts towards reduction and control, are not mutually exclusive. But it is not easy to carry them out simultaneously: they cannot easily be realized as a simultaneous whole.[2] Thus a fundamental polarity prevails between the two approaches.

[1] Many modern methods of registration (film, TV, tape-recording) change the immediate situation here considerably: the therapist actually engaged is not the only one concerned with collecting information.

[2] Von Weizsäcker refers to 'ontic' and 'pathic' kinds of knowledge. Sullivan (1953), again, defines the role of the therapist as that of a 'participant observer'. The modes of expression speak for themselves. And yet a point seems to need emphasis. The question is not so much that there are two kinds of attitudes. We are concerned with the hierarchy of forms of responsibility in knowing. The basic dimension of the scale is this: the possibility of controlling something that encounters us – as opposed to being subordinate to what encounters us. As regards the extreme positions, however, it is possible to speak about a polarity, and even a dialectic relation. The period of enlightenment's effort for equality, with its anticipations of solidarity, was necessary, for example, before it was possible to get humanly near enough to the mentally ill even to observe them. Then again, distance of the observed from them was necessary for different types of mental illness to be distinguishable. But aspects of the fundamentally human structure and dynamics of mental disease would never have unfolded for research without a further step: listening to the behaviour of a mentally ill patient as an address and appeal, and the participation that is associated with this. Currently, again, another phase seems to be prevailing in psychiatry: attempts are being made to verify the basic observations thus attained, and this is being done through studies more concerned with measurement, made from a distance on wider groups of patients. The range of concepts, however, contains much of what has been gained in the 'scuffle' with mental illness that characterizes psychotherapy. Relevant examples here are the family study of schizophrenia represented in Finland by Alanen (1964), or Bräutigam's study (1966) in Heidelberg of the schizophrenic's (pre-illness) types of developmental phases.

Erik provides a concrete illustration of this. The picture of his disease constellation was constructed while both the parents and the boy himself were being treated. Yet, in the encounters between the social worker and Erik's mother, even the mildest clarifying questions appeared to interfere with the mother's readiness to open out: this factor made the therapeutic relationship more superficial. Erik's behaviour in play therapy and the content of his games yielded much information about the family constellation. But the game itself had to arise spontaneously, out of the child's own needs, and organically out of the situations in the play therapy. Until the boy's mother had improved in a certain way, had become more stable, certain basic aspects of the constellation could not be brought into the picture. In addition, Erik's potentialities for concentrating on the play therapy and exploring its drama for himself were directly dependent on this improvement in the mother.

II FREUD'S PRINCIPLE OF ABSTINENCE

Notable disturbances of speech development require long-term treatment if genuine results are to be expected. In such cases all forms of curiosity, even scientifically motivated inquiry, must be subservient to the total situation and to the reserve it dictates. There must be patient waiting. Psychoanalysis is only one basic type of long-term therapeutic investigation or investigational therapy. Its originator, Sigmund Freud, gradually reached the clear insight that psychoanalytic therapy must occur in the spirit of abstinence.[1] This applies to all long-term therapy. One must remember the thorniness of the path to improvement, in practice, for both the treated and the treating. Real progress is only possible when there is willingness to endure the absence of immediate relief and satisfaction. The therapist does not behave in accordance with the patient's expectations, nor is the condition alleviated in the way the patient would wish. The patient, for his part, does not fulfil the expectations of the therapist, nor does he fit

[1] 'Analytic treatment should be carried through, as far as is possible, under privation – in a state of abstinence' (S. Freud, 1919).

in with the therapist's various notions about therapeutic improvement.

This is true for therapists working both individually and in teams. The way to improvement is full of surprises, disappointments, setbacks and unexpected advances for both the patients and the therapists. A path like this is inevitable if the disease constellation is to be permitted to draw the team into its challenges, step by step – leading them into the process of transference described in the preceding chapter. Abstinence also implies more than restraint with regard to the wishes and expectations of the patient, the therapist and everyone involved in the struggle for improvement. It also contains a further recognition: improvement cannot be directly based on any knowledge or method. Improvement will be primarily based on those possibilities of life that are latent and concealed in the persons involved in the disease constellation – particularly, of course, in the patient himself. His potentialities for existence are desperately wound up in his symptoms and in the entire constellation he is involved in. The question, then, is not merely one of removing defects or correcting distortions. Quite the contrary, it is precisely by remaining on the edge of the distortions and the involvements – by giving them their opportunity of saying what they have to say – that we are driven into, or rather we reach into, a process of healing with extensive and deep dimensions.

Something of this is implied in the ancient insight of physicians: *natura sanat*, 'nature heals'. Since Freud, however, it has been understood with increasing clarity that nature's more profound healing only occurs when this 'nature' becomes the patient's personal possession – when he has accepted it and allowed it to emerge in himself and as himself. Nature heals when man has allowed nature to come into being as himself. One immediate practical conclusion from this is the following. In cases of disturbed speech development, one must leave to the children's parents as much personal responsibility for the struggle towards improvement as they can possibly bear – neither more nor less, if one can achieve it. One might express it thus: there is no call to remove from the patient and his parents, and transfer to the team, more of the responsibility than is absolutely necessary. More: there is no reason to try to carry through the diagnostic or elucidative work entirely regardless of the amount of motivation and responsibility to be found in the patient's situation.

In the first roughly orientative examination, some kind of picture is obtained of the child's speech defect. Perhaps, too, one may even form some idea about the defect's actual background in the state of the child's personality. At the same time, one is already in the midst of the phenomenon of 'bringing for treatment'. The quality of this experience is an essential element in the diagnosis and is the beginning of the prognostics. What are the routes that have led the child into this situation of examination? What role are the parents playing here? Who wants an unravelling to take place, and how firmly? Why is help being sought, and primarily for whose needs? Is the pertinent circumstance, perhaps, a desire to get rid of the nuisance, or even the child himself? All in all, at this initial stage, a preliminary impression may be obtained of how stable the investigational and therapeutic constellation is going to be. Sometimes the team's preparedness for abstinence may be immediately put to the test. And a further point can be most significant for the entire development of the therapy: is it going to be possible to ward off a completely inappropriate transfer of responsibility? One might speculate, for instance, about what would have happened if Lauri had been received into treatment under different preconditions. As it was, he was received for treatment under special arrangements due to pressure by the mother. Her main argument was the father's approaching promotion ceremony. What would have happened if the pressure she was applying had been opposed, discussed or even analysed in some way? Or if a prerequisite for the boy's examination had been an encounter with both the parents? Perhaps a more solid foundation for the future disentanglement would have been created than was actually laid. It is by no means easy to settle attitudes in situations like these. It is particularly difficult when the team has already encountered the child and become directly subject to his appeal.

III THE ANTHROPOLOGICAL
STRUCTURE OF THE THERAPEUTIC TASK

Speech therapy – treatment that concentrates on overcoming the speech impediment itself – has hardly been mentioned at all in this study. The need for speech therapy is self-evident: there is no need for it to be underlined. However, a few general considerations are relevant here. Supposing a child who has been brought for examination, owing to a disturbance in speech development, is revealed to be oligophrenic. An attempt should then be made to elucidate the kind of patient he is, in addition to investigating how many capacities he lacks. One must get to know what kind of presence the patient has in both his family and the other communities close to him. Only in such a framework can the teaching of speech performance take its own fully meaningful and sometimes decisively significant place.[1] Mutism, or the abandonment of speech, echolalia, or the autistic use of a private language – these are situations where speech contact and integration are interrupted at a point outside the speech performance itself: in the terrain of the basic prerequisites for speech, in fact. With aphasias of children, concentration on the teaching of speech itself may constitute a natural mode of therapeutic encounter. In this case, however, the teaching event itself becomes a therapeutic process, with extensive dimensions. The teaching has all the problems and requirements characteristic of long-term therapies (such as psychoanalysis). In this respect, for instance, the case of childhood aphasia reported by Landau et al. (1960) is comparable to the history of Helen Keller and Anne Sullivan. The matter can be put thus: the more severe the degree of speech disturbance, the more firmly will speech therapy become part of the total therapy.

In severe cases of disturbance of speech development – where the speech defects are relevant to the child's development and future in general – the parents always constitute a central front for disentanglement and treatment. Unless the parents are taken

[1] Siltala (1964) has illustrated the essence, significance, and position of psychotherapy in the therapeutic entity, where speech impediments are concerned. She has done so substantially and from many aspects.

into account, unless their responsibility becomes productively mobilized, the major part of the team's efforts will easily drain away into futility. The minimum requirement is that there must be some essential point of contact between the nature of the parent's motivation and the team's investigational and therapeutic response. Otherwise, even a multidimensional disentanglement, involving a wealth of well-founded documents and the most ingenious therapeutic methods, may still miss the essential target. Speech therapy may produce the most amazing achievements, though the child only employs his new abilities in contacts with the clinic and in similar specific contexts. The more helpless the prospective patient is, in terms of age, developmental stage, or defectiveness, the more directly the success of the diagnosis and treatment depends on the success on the parental front.

The constellation may demand the most diversified work with the child's parents. Reality here is truly often more baffling than any fairy-tale. It is by no means rare to find onself immediately in the middle of a chaotic marital drama. Sometimes again the parents need guidance on how to obtain the most elementary and available kinds of social care; on how to ward off acute economic distress; or on how, perhaps, therapeutic co-operation can be facilitated despite long distances between home and hospital. This too can require even extensive mediatory work between welfare officers and the parents – if, for example, the situation contains a feature that is new or strange to the officials, or if there is a hole in legislation at this point. As Aatto Sonninen has often pointed out, the designation put on the child's complaint – whether it places him within the sphere of responsibility of the Ministry of Education, the Home Office, or the Ministry of Health, for example – can be crucial for the child's future. Frequently the most immediate task involves encouragement of the parents and their arousal from apathy, for they may be close to fundamental resignation. The broken self-esteem of the parents, the associated paralysis of initiative, and their lack of independence from their own parents or parents-in-law, may often be the first therapeutic obstacle. In some contexts, almost the entire team may come to experience these aspects of the constellation, although the particular task of talking with the parents is often entrusted to the social worker, the psychologist, or some of the doctors – frequently to each of them at different stages of the treatment. In many cases, work with the patient's mother or father (or with the person who fulfils their functional role) assumes the character of prolonged psychotherapy or may lead the person himself to seek such therapy.

Sometimes co-operation with the parents is almost impossible from the very beginning, due to some community factor that can be felt in the background but is only revealed gradually. Perhaps it is gross unsolidarity in some particularly unintegrated village community, involving severe discrimination against the defect; this was the case, for instance, with Pentti, as was revealed in the later stages of Pentti's therapy. In such a case, real contact with the parents is only possible after the team has become aware of the extent of the parent's distress. The nature of this may be only dimly recognized even by the parents themselves. Until the team has begun to see the situation from this point of view, the team's astonishment, perhaps stupefaction, at the parent's apathetic indifference can easily contain elements of implicit accusation – which, in turn, will soon lead to a dead-end situation. Moreover, the team will only be able to identify such distresses if it can bear to recognize within itself a degree of participation in the attitudes of the community, perverted though these may be.

The examination and treatment of disturbances of speech development require not only numerous investigational methods and abundant equipment but also a team that lives and moves in rather manifold dimensions. Sonninen (1964, pp. 45–7) has described the team's composition and forms of action. The time-spans are long between, for instance, EEG and play therapy: integration of these has its own many dimensions and is one of the most central tasks of the team. But here we are not merely concerned with dovetailing each member's contribution with those of the other members and the entire therapy; the picture must also organically include the personal immaturity and fragmentation that exist on some dimension for every member of the team; it must include the meagreness, the unrealism, the distortion and the destructiveness in the interrelations between the members. How could it be otherwise? The only essential is this: the challenges from both the patient and the team – with the immaturities, the neuroticisms, and the destructivenesses involved – must be acknowledged and jointly identified as far as possible. Growth into this task will naturally be easier if some of the team's workers have already had experience in long-term personal therapy from the start, as both patient and therapist, or as a member of another such team.

The team, in fact, is the organism that exposes itself to the second transfer or transference:[1] in this the disease constellations are transferred into the team to become the team's own. Reception of a defective child means assumption of his constellations. The elements that form the problems of the constellation find a representation in the members of the team and in the team's mutual relations. The problems are those which the community has transferred on to the individual child. Here they obtain entry into the organism formed by the team. Problems are thus being transferred back from the child's situation into the community, for the team delegated by the community represents – in a sense is – the community. The types of problems concerned here include the following: opinions and attitudes perverted over generations; human relationships saturated with suspicion; hatred and resentment; relations involving possession, oppression exploitation and submission to the condition of an object; the most varied doctrines of despair; discriminatory practices; and so on. Under various names, or without names, or in the guise of institutionalized traditions, they now penetrate into the team, creating situations between its members.

The team cannot, therefore, easily avoid becoming involved in its task; the team cannot remain outside the turmoil, if, as a whole, it opens itself up to the challenges of disease constellations. It must then willy-nilly become a vicarious field of conflict for the turmoils of disease. According to Erikson (1958a), this constitutes, for the patient, a 'moratorium'. The concept of the moratorium

[1] See the preceding chapter.

designates an opportunity for the special clarification and maturation that the individual needs in his personality crises: the requirement is, in many cases, a time and place for therapy. An adult or adolescent human being is often, partly unconsciously, seeking just such an opportunity through his attitudes; or it is being sought for him by his psychosis, his neurosis, or his psychopathic-asocial distortion. A speech impediment or a child's disturbance of speech development can also constitute such a search. A team that agrees to receive such a person, grant a moratorium and prepare the framework, becomes involved in an intensive process and is challenged to continuous development and human growth. The team has no other choice – unless it rejects the address, refuses to submit to it, and closes its ears, eyes, and entire being. It may, of course, try to remain uninvolved, external, detached, by building some would-be autonomous island for its protection: it might, for example, propose a certain kind of overall scientific programme and attitude for such a purpose. But rejection and denial of this sort can have destructive consequences for the team. The problems about to be transferred, the turmoil now concealed by this very unrecognition, may succeed in penetrating the human structures of the team, but now chaotically and destructively. The disruption, fragmentation, and consequent hardening into division may not be observed at all, however. Instead, even extremely destructive events and processes in the team may be ascribed to 'accident' or, perhaps, to character deficiencies in individual members of the team.

As long as the team as an entity is only dimly aware of the nature of its work – that is, of being a vicarious battlefield – the team experiences the unpalatable elements of therapy as primarily 'caused' by, say, the play therapy or the psychotherapeutic activity in general. These are blamed accordingly. As mentioned in the preceding chapter, it is often precisely in the play therapy that the total therapeutic process culminates. The phases of the internal drama of play therapy are, indeed, to be variously felt in the everyday life of a phoniatric ward. The child's behaviour frequently becomes very unmanageable; sometimes it may even become dangerous for the patient himself or other children. There is actual distress for the therapeutic personnel here, and, in considering it, certain other facts can easily be forgotten:

1 During a healing process the real dangers of the child's constellation will always be encountered in density: the intangible danger, the developmental danger, receives, as it were, concrete form. The question really is one of life and death. Correspondingly, by its very essence, the treatment must in some of its phases necessarily be a walk on a razor's edge.

2 Play therapy is, in fact, specifically psychotherapy; but so – in a way – is the work of the team in general. Play therapy merely constitutes an especially intimate, dually concentrated systematic field of transference. Nevertheless, the entire treatment is the preparation of a moratorium for the patient. It is an attempt to unearth and encourage the potentialities for life that are latent in the constellation and particularly in the child–patient. The treatment thus exists as a field for growth and a battlefield. Actually, this therapeutic whole is usually what the word psychotherapy designates, even if those using the word sometimes think they are only referring to a certain method of therapy or a way of thinking.

In a considerable area of severe disturbance of speech development, psychotherapy, in the special sense of the word, is also required: both as the necessary play therapy and as manifold forms of 'conversational therapy' with the child's parents or their substitutes. For this, sometimes a continuous investment of work lasting as long as several years is required. Only in exceptional cases should the child be kept hospitalized for so long, but sometimes even this cannot be avoided. Such an investment of work, time, effort, and economic resources in a single case of disturbed speech development may appear surprising, even open to question. The decisive factor here, however, is the perspective from which the matter is surveyed. If we are participating, stage by stage, in the therapeutic process of transference, we shall certainly not readily experience the interruption of therapy at some particular stage as natural or even justified 'because the contribution is already adequate and may soon be excessive'. It seems natural to let the actual therapeutic challenges determine whether treatment be continued or not. On the other hand, there are often conflicts because some patients and challenges are being left aside while others are receiving our full efforts. This is a real problem, although it is often mooted without sufficient consideration. There is no easy solution in sight for a dilemma of this nature, for the people involved would not be satisfied for long with a superficial measure: they would not be willing to supply provisional and trivial aid – to some extent merely ostensible aid – to a large number of people, simply because 'there is not enough time, personnel, or means' for devotion to an *authentic* process which is close to the *genuine* challenges.

Factors included and encountered in the structure of such a conflict are our basic conceptions concerning man and disease. These conceptions, after all, guide the decisions we make concerning research and therapeutic institutions and practices. These are the conceptions that have prevailed among us and to which we still give allegiance, and they largely determine the framework for our actions; a framework where we either have, or have not, time, personnel, and means. These structures are essentially formed from our valuations, from what we consider significant, important, or, in general, real. For example, it is possible that only the investigation and treatment that gives an immediate alleviation of speech impairment will be considered to warrant the expense of national funds. Yet there are other considerations. How far has an atmosphere of hope and tolerance arisen in a patient's constellation? How far can the chronic toxicity of a constellation be overcome? These questions may not only be significant in themselves: they may be decisive from an economic point of view as well, leading to unexpected increases in human productivity. Sometimes *this* may be the most substantial result of a long therapeutic struggle, the patient's speech impediment perhaps persisting to a quite considerable degree. Nevertheless, some vicious circle has been broken: perhaps too the handing-on of a disease constellation has been interrupted. A hindrance to a family's life that has passed on from one generation to another has been arrested and is being eliminated. It would not be a short task to provide statistics for such effects on national economic productivity; but for those participating in investigational and therapeutic teams, and for the patients, the matter often requires no special justification. Explication and scientific verification of such changes is nevertheless, of course, an important task.

Economic saving to the nation also occurs through application of the principle of abstinence. Avoidance, to the greatest possible extent, of inappropriate transmission of responsibility – not carrying coals to Newcastle – avoids work that is merely ostensible and largely wasted effort. In assessing the results, it is also easily forgotten that long-term therapy is an occurrence with wide extensions into the community. The question, after all, is of a battle for integration involving quite a host of people. In point of fact, the large economic investment is by no means confined to a single human being. On the contrary, via one individual it has become possible to involve real, shared, socially widespread, and influential disease constellations in treatment. Nor should one underestimate an important 'side-effect' of the therapeutic work: the training of the team itself, their human growth and enrichment, with future therapeutic consequences.

Thus, the tensions and turmoils that arise in the team do belong to the examination, investigation, and treatment themselves; they are not merely 'conditions', or peripheral, secondary nuisances. These pressures must be jointly received and analysed, where this is possible and appropriate; they must be suffered through with shared responsibility; and these tasks constitute an organic part of the investigation and treatment. During this process, important diagnostic clues about the constellation are obtained, and the constellation's transference into the team is identified. Freud originally experienced the phenomenon he later termed transference as an annoying complication of the analytic treatment of neuroses. Gradually, however, he recognized that this same transference was the most central dimension of the treatment itself. This obviously also applies, *mutatis mutandis*, to the investigation and treatment of disturbances of speech development. Here the reception and conduct of transference are by no means limited to the individual psychotherapeutic situations. Transference reveals itself as a particular task and intrinsic process of the team. As far as Sonninen's team is concerned, the team broke down to some extent due to precisely these problems. But a contributory element in this disintegration was that, as a pioneer group in its field, it had only meagre support in the general medical and institutional consciousness. The three-year experience of this process is now assisting the members to participate in the formation of new teams: the nature and extent of the task and difficulties are now many degrees clearer.

The present study has been an analysis of those aspects of the team's investigational and therapeutic experiences that have for me already taken on the outline of a comprehensive picture. I intend to return to certain groups of problems related to disturbance of speech development later. Here, indeed, the problems have been dealt with from the most general points of view possible, without dwelling exhaustively on the problems raised by any particular group of phenomena. I have attempted to define the nature of the problems encountered in my contributory task as a team-member, and I have done so from the point of view of the conception of man that now appears to be – silently and implicitly – emerging in medical science. The central categorical relations of many traditional findings have seemed to acquire a new perspective from the experiences gained within the framework of what is, in some respects, a new type of therapeutic total attitude. A critical analysis of the usage of certain basic medical concepts seemed warranted, for certain concepts of a new type seem to be emerging from contemporary investigational and therapeutic experience.

My task has been to articulate consciously part of the process of metamorphosis that is currently taking place in the medical and scientific conceptions of man and disease.

References

ALANEN, Y. O. 1964. Psykodynamiska familjeundersökningar och deras inverkan på psykiatriska tänkesätt. *Nord. Psykiatr. Tdskft.*, **18**, 409.

ARNOLD, G. E. 1960. Studies in Tachyphemia. *Logos*, **3**, 25.

ASTRADA, C., BAUCH, K., BINSWANGER, L., HEISS, R., KUNZ, H., RUPRECHT, E., SCHADEWALDT, W., SCHREY, H.-H., STAIGER, E., SZILASI, W. & VON WEIZSÄCKER, C. F. 1949. *Martin Heideggers Einfluss auf die Wissenschaften*. Bern: Francke.

BALLY, G. 1959. Das Diagnoseproblem in der Psychotherapie. *Nervenarzt*, **30**, 481.

—— 1961. *Einführung in die Psychoanalyse Sigmund Freuds*. München: Rowohlt.

BINSWANGER, L. 1936. *Freuds Auffassung des Menschen im Lichte der Anthropologie*. New edition 1947 in *Ausgewählte Vorträge und Aufsätze*, Vol. I. Bern: Francke.

BONNHOEFFER, D. 1952. *Widerstand und Ergebung*. München: Kaiser.

BOSS, M. 1954. *Psychosomatische Medizin*. Bern: H. Huber.

BOWLBY, J. 1951. La séparation précoce. *Psychiatrie Soc. de l'Enfance*. Centre Intern. de l'Enfance. Travaux et docum. II, Paris, 45.

BRAUTIGAM, W. 1966. Erlebnisvorfeld und Anlässe schizophrener Psychosen. Paper delivered at a meeting of the Finnish Psychiatric Association.

COOPER, D. 1967. *Psychiatry and Anti-Psychiatry*. London: Tavistock.

ERIKSON, E. H. 1958a. *Childhood and Society*. New York: Norton.

—— 1958b. *Young Man Luther*. New York: Norton.

FOUCAULT, M. 1967. *Madness and Civilization*. London: Tavistock; New York: Pantheon.

FREUD. A. 1965. *Normality and Pathology in Childhood – Assessments of Development*. New York: Int. Univ. Press.

FREUD. S. 1919. Turnings in the Ways of Psycho-Analytic Therapy. In *Collected Papers*, Vol. II. London: Hogarth Press; New York: Basic Books.

GENDLIN, E. T. 1962. *Experiencing and the Creation of Meaning: A Philosophical and Psychological Approach to the Subjective.* New York: The Free Press.

GOLDSTEIN, K. 1948. *Language and Language Disturbances.* New York: Grune & Stratton. Third edition 1960.

HARDY, W. G. 1956. *Problems of Audition, Perception and Understanding.* Los Angeles: Alexander Graham Bell Assoc. for the Deaf.

HEIDEGGER, M. 1947. *Über den Humanismus.* Frankfurt: Klostermann.

HÜBSCHMANN, W. 1963. Viktor von Weizsäckers Lehre von der Krankheitsentstehung. *Hippokrates*, 349.

KÜTEMEYER, W. 1963. *Die Krankheit in ihrer Menschlichkeit.* Göttingen: Vendenhoeck & Ruprecht.

LAING, R. D. 1960. *The Divided Self.* London: Tavistock.

—— 1961. *Self and Others.* London: Tavistock. Second edition 1969.

LAING, R. D. & ESTERSON, A. 1964. *Sanity, Madness and the Family.* Vol. I. *Families of Schizophrenics.* London: Tavistock.

LAING, R. D., PHILLIPSON, H. & LEE, A. R. 1966. *Interpersonal Perception.* London: Tavistock; New York: Springer.

LANDAU, M., GOLDSTEIN, R. & KLEFFNER, F. R. 1960. Congenital Aphasia. *Neurology*, 10.

LE HUCHE, F. 1965. L'exercice du dessin dicté dans le traitement du begaiement. De therapia vocis et loquelae. *Acta Soc. Intern. Logop. Phoniatr.* XIII Congr. Vindobonae, 1, 375.

MACNAB, F. A. 1965. *Estrangement and Relationship.* London: Tavistock; Bloomington, Indiana: Indiana University Press.

MAY, R., ANGEL, E. & ELLENBERGER, H. F. 1958. *Existence, a New Dimension in Psychiatry and Psychology.* New York: Basic Books.

MITSCHERLICH, A. 1969. *Society without the Father.* London: Tavistock; New York: Harcourt Brace.

REENPÄÄ, Y. 1962. *Allgemeine Sinnesphysiologie.* Frankfurt: Klostermann.

RIEBER, R. W. 1965. Word Magic, Self-Alienation and Stuttering. *Folia phoniat.*, 17, 202.

REFERENCES

SIIRALA, A. 1964. *The Voice of Illness.* Philadelphia: The Fortress Press.

SIIRALA, M. 1961. *Die Schizophrenie – des Einzelnen und der Allgemeinheit.* Göttingen: Vanderhoeck & Ruprecht.

—— 1963a. Schizophrenia: A Human Situation. *Amer. J. Psychoanal.*, 23, 39.

—— 1963b. Self-Creating in Therapy. *Amer. J. Psychoanal.*, 23, 164.

—— 1965. On Some Relations Between Thought and Hope. *Acta Philos. Fenn.* 18.

—— Psykiatrinen sairaalayhteisö ja sosiaalipatologia. (The Psychiatric Hospital and Social Pathology.) *Sosiaalilääket. Aik.-L.*, 3, 20.

—— 1966. Our Changing Conception of Illness. *J. Religious Health*, New York, 5.

—— 1966. Peruskatsomustemme merkityksestä lääketieteessä. (Konsultoivan psykiatrin havaintoja puheenkehityksen häiriöistä.) On the Import of our Basic Views in Medicine. (Observations of a consultant psychiatrist on disturbances of speech development.) *Sosiaalilääket, Aik.-L.* Suppl. IIA, Helsinki. (The Finnish version of the present study.)

SILTALA, P. 1964. Psykoterapian osuudesta kielellisissä häiriöissä. (About the Role of Psychotherapy in the Treatment of Speech Disturbances.) *Suom. Logoped. Foniatr. Yhd. julk.*, Helsinki, 5.

SONNINEN, A. 1964. Viivästyneen puheenkehityksen 'q.s. – hypoteesi'. (Quantum satis – Hypothesis in Delayed Speech Development.) *Sosiaalilääket. Aik.-L.*, 2, 41.

SONNINEN, A., SILTALA, P. & SIIRALA, M. 1968. On the Fundamental Prerequisites for Language Development. Report to the XIVth Congress of the International Association of Logopedics and Phoniatrics, Paris.

SPITZ, R. A. 1945. *Hospitalism: An Inquiry into the Genesis of Psychiatric Conditions in Early Childhood. The Psychoanalytic Study of the Child.* New York: International Universities Press; London: Imago.

STRAUSS, E. W. 1966. *Phenomenological Psychology: Selected Papers.* Trans. by E. Eng. New York: Basic Books; London: Tavistock.

SULLIVAN, H. S. 1953. *The Interpersonal Theory of Psychiatry.* New York: Norton.

VON WEIZSÄCKER, V. 1933. *Körpergeschehen und Neurose.* New edition 1947. Stuttgart: Klett.

—— 1940. *Der Gestaltkreis, Theorie der Einheit von Wahrnehmen und Bewegen.* Leipzig.

—— 1951. *Der kranke Mensch.* Stuttgart: Koehler.

—— 1956. *Pathosophie.* Gottingen: Vandenhoeck & Ruprecht.

Index

161

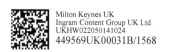